SUBSTANCE ABUSE ASSESSMENT, INTERVENTIONS AND TREATMENT

SUBSTANCE ABUSE

TREATMENT PLANS AND SOBER LIVING HOMES

SUBSTANCE ABUSE ASSESSMENT, INTERVENTIONS AND TREATMENT

Additional books and e-books in this series can be found on Nova's website under the Series tab.

SUBSTANCE ABUSE ASSESSMENT, INTERVENTIONS AND TREATMENT

SUBSTANCE ABUSE

TREATMENT PLANS AND SOBER LIVING HOMES

CAROLINE A. NILSSON
EDITOR

snova
New York

NOTICE TO THE READER

Library of Congress Cataloging-in-Publication Data

ISBN: 978-1-53617-806-7

Published by Nova Science Publishers, Inc. † New York

CONTENTS

PREFACE

In 2015, 20.8 million people aged 12 years or older (7.8 percent of the United States population) had a substance use disorder (SUD) in the previous year. Approximately 75 percent of this group, or 15.7 million Americans, had an alcohol use disorder, 2.0 million had a prescription opioid use disorder (OUD), and about 0.6 million had a heroin use disorder. Even though evidence-based SUD treatments are effective, rates of treatment receipt are quite low. Only about 48 percent of patients who enter SUD treatment actually complete it. One measure of treatment receipt is the Initiation and Engagement of Alcohol and Other Drug Dependence Treatment (IET) performance measure, which is commonly reported by health plans and used by health systems and Medicaid and Medicare programs .Chapter 1 examines how these factors affect health plan performance on the IET measures for both commercial and Medicaid health plans and how initiation and engagement may be improved.

According to the Centers for Disease Control, more than 115 people in the U.S. die after overdosing on opioids every day. In 2017, more than 72,000 Americans died from drug overdoses, overall. It is clear that we need safe and effective recovery options to combat this epidemic to ensure that people have the opportunity to get the help they need. One popular option is known as a sober living home as discussed in chapter 2.

In: Substance Abuse
Editor: Caroline A. Nilsson

ISBN: 978-1-53617-806-7

Chapter 1

BEST PRACTICES AND BARRIERS TO ENGAGING PEOPLE WITH SUBSTANCE USE DISORDERS IN TREATMENT*

Peggy O'Brien, Erika Crable, Catherine Fullerton and Lauren Hughey

OFFICE OF THE ASSISTANT SECRETARY FOR PLANNING AND EVALUATION

The Office of the Assistant Secretary for Planning and Evaluation (ASPE) is the principal advisor to the Secretary of the Department of Health and Human Services (HHS) on policy development issues, and is responsible for major activities in the areas of legislative and budget development, strategic planning, policy research and evaluation, and economic analysis.

---

* This is an edited, reformatted and augmented version of U.S. Department of Health and Human Services Assistant Secretary for Planning and Evaluation Office of Disability, Aging and Long-Term Care Policy, dated March 2019.

ASPE develops or reviews issues from the viewpoint of the Secretary, providing a perspective that is broader in scope than the specific focus of the various operating agencies. ASPE also works closely with the HHS operating agencies. It assists these agencies in developing policies, and planning policy research, evaluation and data collection within broad HHS and administration initiatives. ASPE often serves a coordinating role for crosscutting policy and administrative activities.

ASPE plans and conducts evaluations and research – both in-house and through support of projects by external researchers – of current and proposed programs and topics of particular interest to the Secretary, the Administration and the Congress.

Office of Disability, Aging and Long-Term Care Policy

The Office of Disability, Aging and Long-Term Care Policy (DALTCP), within ASPE, is responsible for the development, coordination, analysis, research and evaluation of HHS policies and programs which support the independence, health and long-term care of persons with disabilities – children, working aging adults, and older persons. DALTCP is also responsible for policy coordination and research to promote the economic and social well-being of the elderly.

In particular, DALTCP addresses policies concerning: nursing home and community-based services, informal caregiving, the integration of acute and long-term care, Medicare post-acute services and home care, managed care for people with disabilities, long-term rehabilitation services, children's disability, and linkages between employment and health policies. These activities are carried out through policy planning, policy and program analysis, regulatory reviews, formulation of legislative proposals, policy research, evaluation and data planning.

The opinions and views expressed in this chapter are those of the authors. They do not reflect the views of the Department of Health and

Human Services, the contractor or any other funding organization. This chapter was completed and submitted on September 29, 2017.

Executive Summary

Background

In 2015, 20.8 million people aged 12 years or older (7.8 percent of the United States population) had a substance use disorder (SUD) in the previous year [1]. Approximately 75 percent of this group, or 15.7 million Americans, had an alcohol use disorder [1], 2.0 million had a prescription opioid use disorder (OUD) [2], and about 0.6 million had a heroin use disorder [1]. Since 1999, opioid-related overdose deaths in the United States have quadrupled, with more than 15,000 individuals experiencing prescription drug-related overdose deaths in 2015 [3]. Even though evidence-based SUD treatments are effective, rates of treatment receipt are quite low. In 2015, only 18 percent of the population with SUDs, or 3.7 million people, received SUD treatment – a number that has not increased significantly since 2002 [1, 4]. Only about 48 percent of patients who enter SUD treatment actually complete it [5].

SUD Treatment Access

In 2015, only 18% of the population with SUDs received treatment – a number that has not increased significantly since 2002. For the definition of SUD and other key terms, see Table A.1. Glossary of terms and definitions. Terms and Definitions.

One measure of treatment receipt is the Initiation and Engagement of Alcohol and Other Drug Dependence Treatment (IET) performance measure, which is commonly reported by health plans and used by health systems and Medicaid and Medicare programs. Reported rates of initiation and engagement vary significantly among health plans, and national rates of initiation and engagement have not improved over time. This variation indicates that some plans are more effective than others at initiating and engaging their members in SUD treatment [6].

In response to the stagnating rates of initiation and engagement, the U.S. Department of Health and Human Services Office of the Assistant Secretary for Planning and Evaluation initiated a study to determine how higher-performing health plans improve initiation and subsequent engagement in SUD treatment. Previous research has shown that many variables may contribute to patients' initiation and engagement in treatment, including individual, provider, health plan, and market and environmental factors. This study examines how these factors affect health plan performance on the IET measures for both commercial and Medicaid health plans and how initiation and engagement may be improved.

Study Objectives and Hypotheses

This study has two overarching objectives:

- Determine the models of care, quality improvement interventions, and best practices used by higher-performing health plans to improve initiation and engagement in SUD treatment.
- Describe the provider, beneficiary, and market factors that affect their ability to successfully initiate and engage beneficiaries in substance use treatment services.

On the basis of existing literature, the research team hypothesized that health plans that performed well on the IET measures would be highly integrated behavioral and physical health service models; they would reimburse for a variety of substance use treatment-related services including case management, routine outreach, peer supports, outpatient, inpatient, partial hospitalization, and residential treatment; they would have high network adequacy and provide financial incentives for providers; and they might be more likely to serve smaller markets in a community-oriented model rather than be plans with large beneficiary enrollment covering diverse populations and geographic areas.

METHODOLOGY

To determine factors that contribute to health plan success in engaging plan members in SUD treatment, we used a sequential, explanatory mixed methods study design where quantitative data were analyzed before qualitative data were collected, to help explain results observed in the quantitative analyses. We initially conducted an environmental scan to provide background on: (1) the epidemiology of substance use, SUDs, and treatment; (2) factors associated with treatment initiation and engagement; (3) interventions designed to improve initiation and engagement; and (4) the development and use of the IET measure. The results of the scan informed both the quantitative and qualitative research that followed.

Initiation and Engagement

We used the NCQA measure of IET in much of this study to define and measure initiation and engagement, which are two separate rates within the measure. A simplified definition of *initiation* is the percentage of members with an alcohol or other drug diagnosis who had at least one instance of treatment within 14 days of diagnosis. *Engagement* is the percentage of members who initiated and had at least two additional substance use treatment visits within 30 days of initiation.

For the quantitative analysis of factors associated with initiation and engagement among adults, we used the 2013 and 2014 Truven Health MarketScan® Commercial Claims and Encounters Research Database, linked to geographic information that provided state-level market characteristics.

The unit of analysis for this study was the employer health plan. We analyzed initiation and engagement rates for SUD treatment and for OUD treatment. We included 321 health plans in our analysis of the rates for SUD treatment, with a mean of 50,585 beneficiaries, and 82 plans for the analysis of the rates for OUD treatment, with a mean of 92,521 beneficiaries. Covariates examined in the quantitative analyses included those related to: (1) health plan structure; (2) reimbursement factors; (3) benefit design; (4) beneficiary characteristics aggregated to the plan level; and (5) state-level market and environmental characteristics. We calculated descriptive statistics separately, and we completed four multivariate regressions to examine the relationship between the selected covariates and the initiation and engagement measure outcomes. Separate analyses addressed initiation and engagement measure outcomes for SUD treatment and for OUD treatment.

For the qualitative research component, we selected potential health plans to study through interviews of their representatives. We chose these plans on the basis of their performance on IET and other behavioral health measures reported in National Committee for Quality Assurance (NCQA) Quality Compass data for commercial plan performance from January 1, 2015, through December 31, 2015, and for Medicaid plan performance from January 1, 2014, through December 31, 2014. The NCQA Healthcare Effectiveness Data and Information Set measure data capture at least 75 percent of health plans in the United States. Outreach to top-ranked plans resulted in six site visits – one with a commercial plan and five with Medicaid plans.

To guide the health plan interviews, we developed a site visit protocol and semi-structured discussion guide. Research team members conducted qualitative, semi-structured group interviews with health plan staff and affiliates in spring 2017. Interviews were analyzed using a thematic framework analysis approach in combination with more inductive strategies to enable novel themes to emerge within the analysis.

Quantitative Results

The quantitative multivariate analyses indicated that, among other findings, higher rates of SUD treatment initiation were associated with providing higher numbers of intensive outpatient (IOP) and partial hospitalization services per beneficiary ($\beta = 2.06408$, $p = 0.0103$). Results also suggested that having higher out-of-pocket costs for outpatient SUD services per user may be associated with higher rates of SUD initiation per beneficiary ($\beta = 0.000517$, $p = 0.0007$). Higher rates of SUD engagement were associated with similar characteristics, specifically providing higher numbers of IOP and partial hospitalization services per beneficiary ($\beta = 3.82326$, $p < 0.0001$) and higher numbers of SUD outpatient services per beneficiary ($\beta = 4.13869$, $p < 0.0001$). Higher rates of engagement were negatively associated with having more beneficiaries in the plan with an identified SUD ($\beta = -12.6598$, $p = 0.0001$) and more beneficiaries who are female ($\beta = -0.20293$, $p = 0.0497$).

Characteristics associated with higher rates of initiation of OUD treatment included providing higher numbers of IOP and partial hospitalization services per beneficiary ($\beta = 4.47344$, $p = 0.0409$) and being in a state with a higher prevalence of opioid prescriptions relative to the state population ($\beta = 0.00228$, $p = 0.024$). Higher rates of engagement were associated with providing higher numbers of SUD IOP and partial hospitalization services per beneficiary ($\beta = 4.07017$, $p = 0.0001$). Higher engagement was negatively associated with, for example, having a higher percentage of beneficiaries with an identified OUD ($\beta = -10.549$, $p = 0.0089$) or a higher percentage of beneficiaries who are female ($\beta = -0.1958$, $p = 0.0233$).

Qualitative Results

Representatives from six health plans participated in interviews. The plans served geographically diverse populations across the United States, and all were ranked in the top 5 percent (nationally) for performance on initiation and/or engagement rates using the IET measure. The intent was to have a mix of commercial and Medicaid plans; ultimately representatives from one commercial and five Medicaid plans participated in the study.

Health Plan Structure

Some level of local decision-making is critical to implementing behavioral health policies and procedures in ways that respond to local population needs, whether the plan is small and local or large and national.

Governance and Structure

Our interviews included representatives of large and small health plans. Representatives of smaller, locally governed plans described the importance of a "feet on the street" approach, whereas interviewees from a national insurance company with a centralized corporate leadership felt that their approach enabled them to streamline decision-making and ensure consistency across business lines. For all but the smallest plan, however, interviewees typically described a multilevel governance approach, including corporate and local oversight of behavioral health care, although the extent of plan emphasis on local governance represented a spectrum. Because these were all higher-performing plans, it is impossible to determine whether one approach more consistently translates into improved initiation or engagement. A locally focused approach may be one of the ways that the selected plans differentiate themselves from others that may fare more poorly on initiation and engagement, if lack of local governance and local initiatives are more limited among the latter. Interviewees also highlighted the importance of regular communication between plan levels and between different groups within plan levels regarding beneficiary needs or challenges to accessing health services.

Care Model and Culture

Interviewees from every health plan described their plan's care model and culture as integral to their success with initiating and engaging beneficiaries in treatment. Care models were described as focused on care coordination, including coordination of physical, mental, behavioral, and substance-use-specific services. All health plan representatives described their case managers, care coordinators, and community health workers as promoting beneficiaries' use of services included within the plan's benefit array.

Health plan leadership and contracting staff also described efforts to convey the health plan's mission statement when meeting with new providers to reinforce the plans' commitment to continuous engagement with beneficiaries, knowing that beneficiary receptiveness will vary over time.

Benefit Design

Health plan interviewees described significant differences in their plan benefit arrays. All plans cover outpatient treatment services without prior authorization. All cover medically monitored and medically managed detoxification services, often requiring prior authorization or notification, but one only covers these services for pregnant women.

A Role for Prior Notification

Prior notification may play a role in allowing health plans to coordinate care and ensure follow-up after hospitalization or detoxification by alerting the plan to the patient's admission in a timely fashion.

Inpatient, IOP, and partial hospitalization services frequently require prior authorization. Coverage of peer and recovery support services was sparse among Medicaid plans. The commercial plan provides members access to peer supports as part of their "service buffet" offered at all affiliate SUD treatment clinics. All health plans provide members with coverage of at least two medication-assisted treatment (MAT) options and cover naloxone. Most representatives do not require prior authorization for MAT.

Representatives of Medicaid plans described limitations on their ability to reimburse for residential treatment services because of state Medicaid policy, with four of the five interviewees indicating that their (four separate) state Medicaid agencies did not include residential treatment in Medicaid benefits for non-pregnant beneficiaries. The one Medicaid plan with a residential treatment benefit was able to approve only limited residential services. Conversely, the commercial plan reported residential services as a covered benefit.

None of the Medicaid plans required beneficiaries to pay for covered services out-of-pocket. The commercial plan representative described their benefit array as an "all you can eat buffet" of services, free of prior authorization or utilization management review but requiring payment of a deductible.

Quality Improvement

Health plan interviewees reported investing significant resources in quality improvement activities, expressing a concern that poorly managed SUDs would result in higher overall costs for the plan as well as inadequate care for beneficiaries. Quality improvement efforts include developing new staff positions to support activities, investing in software to develop data analytic capabilities, and facilitating secure communications with beneficiaries and providers. To maximize returns, two of the Medicaid plans reported focusing their time and financial investments on initiatives that targeted activities related to quality measures for which they were financially at risk under the state Medicaid plan. Types of quality improvement initiatives vary, in part because of the different levels of resources available to plans.

All representatives described open communication within the plan and between the plan and their membership or providers as key to achieving improvements in SUD treatment.

Communication strategies included using secure electronic messaging services to maintain real-time communication with providers. Outreach teams are trained on effective communication techniques to encourage members to engage in treatment. Health plan interviewees expressed a substantial interest in maintaining communication between physical health and behavioral health providers. Some interviewees also described co-locating behavioral health counselors in primary care practices as critical to treatment initiation for patients who would not attend services provided in a behavioral health facility.

Health Plan Members at Moderate Risk of SUD

Health plans are increasingly using data analytics to identify members misusing opioid prescriptions, enabling outreach to and treatment for individuals who may not have any previous indicator of risk.

Barriers Affecting Health Plan Initiation and Engagement Rates

Health plan interviewees described several factors that influence their plans' effectiveness at initiating and engaging members in substance use treatment services.

Federal and state policies were identified as major factors affecting health plans' ability to provide comprehensive services to meet membership needs. Interviewees described federal confidentiality requirements of 42 Code of Federal Regulations (CFR) Part 2 as challenging to coordinating care for members admitted to detox and other inpatient facilities. Health plan stakeholders described learning of beneficiary detox admissions only after the beneficiary had been discharged. Another federal policy they mentioned was the restriction on Medicaid coverage of care in Institutions for Mental Diseases (IMD), which precludes Medicaid reimbursement for residential facilities with more than 15 beds, although some states are obtaining Section 1115 waivers to allow reimbursement for residential care.

Representatives from each of the five Medicaid plans also identified policies emanating from their state Medicaid agency as factors limiting their ability to initiate and engage members in SUD treatment. They viewed restrictions on the types of services included in the state Medicaid benefit array, such as for residential treatment or peer and recovery supports, as a substantial barrier. Some expressed a desire to cover additional treatment services not reimbursable by the state, but ultimately felt doing so was beyond their financial capabilities.

Medicaid plan representatives said that state Medicaid policies allowing beneficiaries to switch plans negatively affected their ability to coordinate services or meaningfully use pharmacy or prescriber lock-in programs. A few representatives described placing beneficiaries in lock-in programs to monitor their prescription use while conducting outreach and case management efforts, only to have the beneficiary switch mid-year to another plan. Similarly, plan inability to access Prescription Drug Monitoring Program (PDMP) data prevents plans from learning if beneficiaries are evading lock-ins by paying for controlled substances with cash.

All health plan representatives explained that network adequacy for SUD treatment services was a current concern and a major barrier to future access to treatment. Although each of the health plans is meeting network requirements set by the state Medicaid agency and their governance boards, interviewees repeatedly described having additional network needs. First, the growing need for treatment coincides with decreases in the number of substance use providers. Second, there is limited access to Drug Addiction Treatment Act of 2000-waivered buprenorphine prescribers willing to treat Medicaid beneficiaries. Third, prescribers often will not take Medicaid beneficiaries because of preconceived notions about that population, or because they accept only cash for services. Fourth, in addition to reimbursement constraints, there is a lack of beds available in residential treatment facilities. Fifth, low reimbursement rates limit plans' ability to recruit providers to their network and expand network adequacy for necessary services, and ultimately to ensure access to care. Providers withhold open spots from Medicaid beneficiaries to receive greater reimbursement from commercial plans and individuals paying out-of-pocket.

Stigma around substance use and behavioral health treatment repeatedly was cited as a barrier to treatment, hindering effective initiation and engagement. Stigma may manifest in patients, their families, their communities, and providers. Interviewees reported supporting community education about SUDs and the positive impact of treatment as ways to reduce stigma in the community and among those who might need treatment. They also described investing resources in reducing provider stigma related to SUDs. Interviewees also said that providers often hesitate to conduct substance use risk screenings because they had not received adequate addiction training and were uncertain about how to speak with their patients about such issues.

Combating Stigma & Improving Care Coordination

Co-location of SUD counseling and other services with primary care reduces the stigma of accessing a facility identified as treating SUDs, catches members in locations where they are more comfortable, and permits improved coordination between physical and behavioral health care.

Plan members are not always ready to abstain from substance use or other related risk behaviors, which may result in unwillingness to initiate traditional substance use treatment. Health plans are more frequently promoting harm reduction techniques and "no wrong door" and "no wrong time" approaches to engage members in SUD treatment.

Interviewees also described plan members' competing priorities such as housing, child care, and accessing treatment for comorbid physical and behavioral health conditions as factors affecting initiation or engagement in SUD treatment services. They identified beneficiaries who are homeless or transient as challenging to engage because they do not have stable addresses or phone numbers to maintain outreach. They described efforts to provide members with transportation to follow-up appointments as a means of ensuring attendance. Despite being able to offer these supports, case managers indicated that beneficiaries' attendance at follow-up appointments still was impeded by competing demands.

Discussion

The opioid epidemic has worsened a pre-existing failure to provide SUD treatment to many people in the United States who desperately need it. Many of those in need of treatment do not attempt to access it, and many who try find access difficult or impossible. The aim of this study was to determine how some health plans successfully get beneficiaries into SUD treatment and keep them there. Our environmental scan identified many potential influences on initiation and engagement, falling into the four categories of individual, provider, environmental or market, and health plan factors. Our quantitative analyses linking beneficiary, plan, and market characteristics to commercial health plans, as well as subsequent semi-structured interviews with high performing plans, elucidated a variety of key influences, many of which are summarized above.

Individual Influences

The literature indicates that many individual influences can affect initiation and engagement. Among those influences, some, including the individual's sex [7, 8, 9, 10], co-occurring conditions [11], and stigma [12], were addressed in the quantitative or qualitative components of this study. The literature indicates that being female decreases the likelihood of treatment participation [7, 8, 9, 10]. Our quantitative research indicated that plans with larger percentages of females are less likely to do well on the engagement rate, and our qualitative research allowed us to elaborate on why (e.g., competing needs such as child care and transportation). Some successful plans have implemented initiatives designed to address these needs, but effects of these efforts were mixed. The qualitative part of this study also identified ways in which plans seek to better integrate SUD and mental health treatment and to address stigma among patients, families, communities, and providers. It seems that efforts to integrate care, co-locate services, and provide education all can help alleviate stigma and address conditions that co-occur with SUD.

Provider Influences

Consistent with previous research, health plan interviewees reported that provider expertise [13, 14, 15], attitudes [16], and shortages [17, 18, 19] can influence treatment initiation and engagement, and they described steps plans have taken to address problems in these areas.

These include efforts aimed at improving expertise and comfort and decreasing provider stigma about individuals with SUDs. However, at least one plan representative expressed hesitation about developing provider-focused initiatives such as educational activities for fear of overwhelming providers with information on new initiatives, tools, and other SUD-related information. Interestingly, such plans may focus quality improvement efforts more extensively on patients than on providers. Most take both approaches. Within the qualitative sample of only six high performing plans, however, neither approach stood out as particular to the plans with the highest performance.

Efforts to address provider expertise and attitudes should somewhat alleviate provider shortages. Although plan representatives described outreach and other approaches to induce providers into their networks, solving the problem of provider shortages is not simple.

Shortages of individual providers such as addiction specialists, psychiatrists, and buprenorphine prescribers, as well as of residential treatment, detox facilities, or opioid treatment programs, combine to make access to the right level of care at the right time difficult for many plan beneficiaries.

Market and Environmental Influences

The qualitative part of this study most clearly identified market and environmental factors that influence SUD treatment initiation and engagement, some of which are addressed in previous literature. Health plan interviewees identified both federal and state policies that can be barriers to initiation and engagement. The two primary perceived federal impediments were: (1) the regulation at 42 CFR Part 2, which may be met with prior authorization requirements or efforts to build relationships with facilities; and (2) the IMD restriction on reimbursement, which now may be ameliorated with a Section 1115 waiver [20]. State policies that prevent plans from accessing PDMP data or that allow beneficiaries to switch plans easily were seen as impeding the effectiveness of pharmacy lock-ins. State Medicaid plans that do not reimburse for certain services [21, 22], such as peer or recovery supports, or state Medicaid programs with budgetary problems that result in low or delayed reimbursement [18], can impede the ability of Medicaid plans to engage providers and serve their beneficiaries. Plans struggle with the repercussions of these policies, trying to find ways to serve their beneficiaries while accommodating the policy or law.

Health Plan Influences

Health plans take many approaches to improving initiation and engagement in SUD treatment. Health plan structure; benefit design and reimbursement [21, 22, 23, 24, 25]; network adequacy; and the culture of care and approach to care integration, coordination, and management [26, 27] all play roles in how health plans influence initiation and engagement. Quantitative and qualitative analyses identified organizational interventions as factors in increasing treatment uptake. The health plan staff members we interviewed were invested in a variety of quality improvement initiatives at both the enterprise and local plan level, including initiatives with providers and beneficiaries and internal plan initiatives such as data mining and communication strategies. The plans viewed these quality improvement initiatives as important to further treatment access, to improve the quality of care, and, given the high costs that can be associated with undertreated SUDs, to conserve resources.

Implications

This study has many implications, which include the following:

1) Expanding treatment options to cover the care continuum, including peer and recovery specialists, may help provide access to care when it is needed and at the level most relevant to a particular patient. Among other things, expanding Section 1115 waivers to allow Medicaid reimbursement of residential treatment may have the secondary effect of increasing the number of residential placements available for everyone.
2) Finding ways to either modify or provide better education regarding 42 CFR Part 2 could assist plans in their efforts to enhance care coordination and follow-up. Allowing plans access to PDMP data will provide them with better information about their beneficiaries' access to controlled substances.
3) Various aspects of health plan structure such as size, decision locus, and communication strategies play an apparent role in the health plans' ability to ensure treatment initiation and engagement. These same factors also may play a role in follow-up after hospitalization or emergency department visits and in other care coordination efforts. Better understanding of the influence of these factors in lower-performing plans will be important as we move to a health care system that is more coordinated and integrated across settings and disciplines.
4) Making certain that there are mechanisms to pay for care coordination and management, as well as cross-system integration, will be important to improve SUD treatment initiation and engagement.
5) Finding ways to encourage co-location of behavioral and primary care services – where there can be a warm hand-off, where stigma is reduced, and where varied services are close by – will help increase initiation and engagement, as well as integrate SUD treatment into the general health care system.
6) By addressing human needs that compete with treatment, we also may be able to address initiation and engagement differences between men and women, as well as treatment disparities related to socioeconomic differences.

7) By addressing workforce shortages, adequacy of reimbursement, and provider stigma, we may help alleviate some of the provider shortages described in the study. By finding ways to incentivize providers not to require cash payment, additional providers may be brought into payer networks.
8) Researchers and policymakers should consider whether alternative approaches to measuring network adequacy can help maximize health plan networks when provider shortages create an obstacle.
9) When there are financial incentives for health plans, those plans tend to focus quality improvement efforts on the metrics for which they may be paid. This can have repercussions for beneficiary care, and the metrics should be selected carefully.

Study Limitations

Like all studies, this one has limitations. First, the rapid change that has taken place in recent years in health care means that health plans identified for potential interviews on the basis of 2014 results on the IET measure were somewhat different when staff members were interviewed in 2017. Both IET rates and plan strategies for improving SUD treatment participation may have continued, grown, or decreased. Second, the quantitative analyses used commercial insurance data, whereas the qualitative interviews were primarily with Medicaid plans. Although this represents a difference between the quantitative and qualitative aspects of the study, it may provide the benefit of balancing the information gathered. Third, some variables used in the quantitative analyses may not have completely captured the sort of information that was intended. For example, some of the market and environmental variables intended to indicate level of state support for SUD treatment may be an imperfect proxy for market or policy realities.

Conclusion

Identifying mechanisms to enhance SUD treatment initiation and continued engagement in care is a public health priority. As both administrators and coordinators of health care benefits, health plans are positioned to play a crucial role in mitigating potential access barriers and developing mechanisms that bring beneficiaries into care and keep them there. Understanding the role that health plans can play, as well as the role that other factors have in health plans' ability to improve SUD treatment initiation and continued engagement, is important to facilitate improvement in care increasingly reimbursed by these private organizations.

For the reader's convenience, we include a glossary of some terms used in this chapter and a list of common acronyms and abbreviations in Table A.1 and Table A.2.

INTRODUCTION

The 2015 National Survey on Drug Use and Health (NSDUH) found that 20.8 million people aged 12 years or older (7.8 percent of the United States population) had a substance use disorder (SUD) in the previous year [1]. Evidence-based SUD treatments such as behavioral therapies and medication are effective, as evidenced by hundreds of rigorous efficacy trials and millions of individuals in recovery. However, despite the great need for and efficacy of these treatments, rates of treatment receipt are extremely low. In 2015, only 3.7 million people received SUD treatment – a number that has not increased significantly since 2002 [1, 4]. Moreover, once individuals enter treatment, they tend to drop out before obtaining meaningful benefits. Only about 48 percent of patients who enter SUD treatment actually complete it [5], even as research has shown that engagement in treatment improves treatment outcomes [28].

Among other initiatives, one way that federal, state, and privately funded health care systems have tried to address the low rates of initiation and engagement in SUD treatment is through performance metrics. Federal, state, and private payers have incorporated measures endorsed by the National Quality Forum into their programs to track performance among health plans.

One such performance measure is Initiation and Engagement of Alcohol and Other Drug Dependence Treatment (IET).

SUD Treatment Access

In 2015, only 18% of the population with SUD received treatment – a number that has not increased significantly since 2002.

The rate of IET varies significantly among health plans, suggesting that some plans are more effective at initiating and engaging their members in SUD treatment than others [6]. Overall national rates of initiation and engagement have not shown consistent improvement over time. In commercial and Medicaid health plans, respectively, rates for initiation have hovered between 39.1 percent and 49.0 percent, and rates of engagement have stayed between 9.6 percent and 16.2 percent throughout the past decade, with no sustained improvement [29].

In response to the stagnating rates of initiation and engagement, the U.S. Department of Health and Human Services (HHS) Office of the Assistant Secretary for Planning and Evaluation (ASPE) initiated a study to determine how higher-performing health plans improve initiation and subsequent engagement in SUD treatment. This chapter synthesizes the results of quantitative analyses of commercial health plan data and qualitative interviews with Medicaid and commercial plans, to determine health plan and other factors that influence initiation and engagement in SUD treatment. We provide background gleaned from the literature, address the methods for both the quantitative and qualitative analyses, present the results of that research, and offer a synthesis of the findings, including an overview of health plan and related factors that influence initiation and engagement.

Epidemiology of Substance Use and Substance Use Disorders in the United States

Substance use and SUDs are a persistent public health concern. The 2015 NSDUH found that approximately 138.3 million Americans aged 12 years or older reported past 30-day use of alcohol, and 27 million reported past 30-day use of illicit drugs (Table 1) [1]. National prevalence rates also are high for SUDs. Approximately 20.8 million Americans aged 12 years or older were classified with an SUD in 2015. Among those identified, 7.7 million had an illicit drug use disorder; 15.7 million had an alcohol use disorder; and 2.7 million were diagnosed with both an alcohol and an illicit drug SUD (Table 1) [1]. Individuals aged 18-25 years had the highest rates of SUDs in 2015, with 18.2 percent of that age group having an SUD in the past year [2]. A separate study that examined rates of SUDs in older adults estimated that, by 2020, approximately 5.7 million adults aged 50 years and older will have an SUD [30].

Table 1. Summary of 30-day prevalence rates of substance use and annual prevalence rates of dependence or abuse of alcohol and illicit drugs among people aged 12 years and older in 2015

Substance	Use in the Past 30 Days		Dependence or Abuse[a]	
	N (in millions)	% of population	N (in millions)	% of population
Any substance	–	–	20.8	7.8
Alcohol	138.3	51.7	15.7	5.9
Illicit drug	27.1	10.1	7.7	2.9
Alcohol and illicit drug	–	–	2.7	1.0

Source: 2015 NSDUH [1].

[a.] The 2015 NSDUH still used the terms *abuse* and *dependence* rather than the umbrella term *substance use disorder* with gradations of severity that was adopted in the *Diagnostic and Statistical Manual of Mental Disorders, 5th Edition* (DSM-V). Whenever this chapter provides information from the 2015 NSDUH that specifies *abuse* or *dependence*, the report uses those terms. If the NSDUH provided less granular information about disorders generally, this chapter refers to *substance use disorders*.

Epidemiology of Alcohol Use and Alcohol Use Disorders

Alcohol use, including binge drinking and heavy alcohol use, is common in the United States. Approximately 138.3 million Americans aged 12 years or older reported past 30-day use of alcohol in 2015 [1]. Approximately 66.7 million people, or one in four individuals aged 12 years or older in 2015, engaged in past 30-day binge drinking, with binge drinking defined as four or more drinks on one occasion for females and five or more drinks for males [1]. Heavy alcohol use, which is defined as binge drinking on 5 or more days in the past 30 days, was present in an estimated 17.3 million individuals aged 12 years or older, or 6.5 percent of the population, in 2015 [1]. In that same year, approximately 15.7 million Americans had an alcohol use disorder [1].

Table 2. Alcohol use and disorder prevalence in 2015 by selected demographic characteristics

Characteristics	Past 30-Day Alcohol Use, %	Alcohol Use Disorder, %	Binge Drinking, %	Heavy Alcohol Use, %
Age, years				
12-17	9.6	2.5	5.8	0.9
18-25	58.3	10.9	39.0	10.9
26 and older	55.6	5.4	24.8	6.4
Sex				
Male	56.2	7.8	29.6	8.9
Female	47.4	4.1	20.5	4.2
Race/ethnicity				
Non-Hispanic White	57.0	6.1	26.0	7.6
Non-Hispanic Black	43.8	4.9	23.4	4.8
Asian	39.7	3.2	14.0	2.2
Native Hawaiian or other Pacific Islander	33.8	5.4	17.8	3.0
American Indian and Alaska Native	37.9	9.7	24.1	4.7
Two or more races	42.8	6.2	22.9	6.8
Hispanic	42.4	6.4	25.7	4.8

Source: 2015 NSDUH [2].

Alcohol use and alcohol use disorders are more pronounced in certain demographic groups, including individuals aged 18-25 and males, with rates of past-month alcohol use highest in the non-Hispanic White population and alcohol use disorders highest in Native Americans (Table 2) [1]. There also is evidence that women's rates of alcohol use are heavily influenced by pregnancy status. In 2015, approximately 54.8 percent of non-pregnant women of childbearing age (15-44 years old) consumed alcohol in the past month, whereas those who were pregnant had past-month drinking rates of 9.3 percent. Rates were highest (16.4 percent) among those in the first trimester, followed by the second (6.1 percent) and third (4.3 percent) trimesters [2].

Epidemiology of Illicit Drug Use and Illicit Drug Use Disorders

In 2015, approximately 27.1 million Americans reported past 30-day illicit drug use, including those who misused prescription medication. The prevalence rate for past 30-day illicit drug use corresponds to one in every ten Americans or about 10.1 percent of the United States population [1]. Demographic groups with the highest rates of recent illicit drug use included those aged 18-25 years, males, and individuals identifying as being of two or more races (Table 3). Among these groups, there is evidence that women's rates of illicit drug use may be heavily influenced by age. Approximately 12.5 percent of non-pregnant women of childbearing age (15-44 years) engaged in past-month illicit drug use. This percentage was nearly 50 percent higher than the percentage for the female population overall. Approximately 4.7 percent of pregnant women (15-44 years old) reported illicit drug use, with rates highest among those in the second trimester (6.4 percent) [2].

In 2015, 7.7 million Americans had an illicit drug use disorder, constituting nearly 3 percent of the population aged 12 years or older [2]. It is estimated that 9.9 percent of the United States population will develop a drug use disorder at some point during their lifetimes [31]. The highest prevalence rates were in people between the ages of 18 and 25, males, and those identifying as of two or more races (Table 3).

Opioid use and opioid use disorders (OUDs), whether related to heroin or to prescription opioid use, are among the most problematic substance use trends in the United States today. Since 1999, opioid-related overdose deaths in the United States have quadrupled, with more than 15,000 individuals experiencing prescription drug-related overdose deaths in 2015 [3]. Evidence shows that, among those with commercial insurance, professional charges for OUD treatment rose by more than 1,000 percent from 2011 to 2015 (from $71.66 million to $721.80 million).

Total annual charges in 2015 for a person diagnosed with an OUD were 556 percent higher than the average for all patients [32].

Table 3. Illicit drug use and disorder prevalence in 2015 by selected demographic characteristics

Characteristics	Past 30-Day Illicit Drug Use, %	Illicit Drug Use Disorder, %
Age		
12-17 years	8.8	3.4
18-25 years	22.3	7.2
26 years and older	8.2	2.1
Sex		
Male	12.5	3.8
Female	7.9	2.0
Race/ethnicity		
Non-Hispanic White	10.2	2.8
Non-Hispanic Black	12.5	3.5
Asian	4.0	1.2
Native Hawaiian or other Pacific Islander	9.8	4.5
American Indian and Alaska Native	14.2	4.1
Two or more races	17.2	4.9
Hispanic	9.2	3.0

Source: 2015 NSDUH [2].

Heroin Use and Heroin Use Disorders

Rates of heroin use have increased in recent years, from a relatively stable rate of 0.2 percent of the population between 2002 and 2011 to 0.3 percent starting in 2012 (Table 4) [1]. In 2015, approximately 0.3 million Americans aged 12 years and older reported past-month heroin use, and about 828,000 people reported past-year use [1]. The 2015 NSDUH, however, revealed a dramatic reduction in the rate of new heroin users aged 12 years or older. In 2013, an estimated 169,000 individuals began engaging in heroin use in the year prior to being interviewed, and this number increased to 212,000 in 2014. The incidence of new users in 2015, however, decreased to 135,000. Past-year initiation rates also decreased as a percentage of past-year users (24.9 percent in 2013, 23.1 percent in 2014, 16.3 percent in 2015) [2, 33]. Young adults aged 18-25 years are more likely than any other age group to use heroin. In 2015, 0.6 percent of young adults aged 18-25 years reported past-year heroin use [1], with 57,000 initiating heroin use in 2015 [2].

The prevalence of heroin use disorders also has grown in recent years (Table 4). In 2015, about 0.6 million people or 0.2 percent of the population aged 12 years or older had a heroin use disorder in the past year [1]. This was a statistically significant increase from 2010, when 0.1 percent of the population had a heroin use disorder [4]. Young adults were more likely than any other age group to be dependent on heroin (0.4 percent in 2015) [1]. Past-year heroin use disorder prevalence among those aged 18-25 years was 585,000 in 2015 (Table 4) [2]. Among adults aged 26 years and older, the prevalence of heroin dependence or abuse was 430,000 in 2015, or 0.2 percent of the population [2].

Table 4. Percentages of heroin use disorders and past-year heroin use over time

Characteristic	Age, Years	2002	2010	2011	2012	2013	2014	2015
Past-year heroin use	12+	0.2[a]	0.2	0.2	0.3	0.3	0.3	0.3
	18-25	0.4[a]	0.6	0.7	0.8	0.7	0.8	0.6
Heroin use disorder	12+	0.1	0.1	0.2	0.2	0.2	0.2	0.2
	18-25	0.2[a]	0.3	0.4	0.5	0.5	0.5	0.4

Source: 2015 NSDUH [1].

[a.] Significant at the 0.05 level compared with 2015.

Heroin use disorder rates have a strong, positive correlation with heroin-related morbidity and overdose deaths over time [34]. Among individuals with SUDs, heroin users have the highest prevalence of hospitalization (a 30 percent annual rate between 2009 and 2013) [35]. As dependence rates have increased, so have rates of heroin-related overdoses.

There were nearly 13,000 heroin overdose deaths in 2015 [36]. The increase in overdoses has affected individuals across a range of sociodemographic groups. Between 2010 and 2012, heroin-related overdoses increased 86 percent to 102 percent for every age group. In 2012, males had a heroin-related overdose rate of 3.3 per 100,000, which was a 99 percent increase from 2010.

In 2015, males aged 25-44 years had the highest death rates at 13.2 per 100,000 – an increase of 22.2 percent from 2014 [36]. Women experienced a 110.9 percent increase in heroin-related overdoses between 2010 and 2012. Rates of heroin-related overdose also have increased for each racial group in recent years. For both the non-Hispanic White and Hispanic White populations, heroin-related overdoses increased by approximately 102 percent between 2010 and 2012. The African-American community experienced an 89.3 percent increase in heroin-related overdoses for the same time period [37].

Heroin-Related Overdoses

Between 2010 and 2012, heroin-related overdoses increased 86% to 102%.

Prescription Opioid Misuse and Disorders

In 2015, 3.8 million individuals aged 12 years or older in the United States (1.4 percent of the population) reported current misuse (non-medical use) of prescription opioids. The number of individuals who reported past-year prescription opioid misuse was 12.5 million or 4.7 percent of the population. In that year, hydrocodone medications were the most frequently misused category of prescription opioids – misused by 2.7 percent of those aged 12 years or older in 2015 – followed by oxycodone medications (1.6 percent). In 2015, a total of 2.1 million individuals initiated prescription opioid misuse, and 2.0 million individuals had a prescription OUD (both 0.8 percent of those aged 12 years or older) [2]. According to the NSDUH, the demographic groups with the highest prevalence of prescription opioid misuse in 2015 included young adults aged 18-25 years, males, and individuals identified as being two or more races.

The NSDUH did not report rates of prescription OUD other than by age, with those aged 18-25 years having the highest rates of such disorders (Table 5).

Nearly half of all opioid overdose deaths involve a prescription opioid. Such deaths have quadrupled since 1999 and, in 2015, more than 15,000 individuals experienced prescription drug-related overdose deaths [3]. Rudd et al. (2016) examined trends in both heroin and prescription opioid-related overdose death rates across 28 states from 2010 through 2015 [38].

Table 5. Prescription opioid misuse and disorder prevalence in 2015 by selected demographic characteristics

Characteristics	Past 30-Day Prescription Opioid Misuse, %	Prescription OUD, %
Age		
12-17 years	3.9	0.5
18-25 years	8.5	1.2
26 years and older	4.1	0.7
Sex		
Male	5.3	–
Female	4.0	–
Race/ethnicity		
Non-Hispanic White	4.8	–
Non-Hispanic Black	4.4	–
Asian	1.8	–
Native Hawaiian or other Pacific Islander	5.4	–
American Indian and Alaska Native	5.6	–
Two or more races	8.4	–
Hispanic	5.0	–

Source: 2015 NSDUH [2].

Rates of death from synthetic opioids other than methadone increased and, although many of these deaths involved prescription opioids, the increase seems to have been driven by illicitly manufactured fentanyl. In

2015, death rates from non-methadone synthetic opioids were greatest in males aged 25-44 years [38].

Substance Use Disorder Treatment Access and Uptake in the United States

Evidence-based treatment can effectively help people recover from SUDs [39]. Recent analyses indicate that the addition of a single substance abuse treatment facility in a county may be associated with declines in rates of drug-induced mortality and many types of violent and financially motivated crimes, with an additional treatment facility reducing social costs attributed to all crime by approximately $700,000 annually. SUD treatment also has been shown to result in meaningfully reduced rates of crime, with a 10 percent relative increase in the SUD treatment rate at an average cost of $1.6 billion yielding a crime reduction benefit of $2.5-$4.8 billion [40]. Other studies show that, for every dollar spent on SUD treatment, four dollars are saved in other health care costs [12].

Many Americans in need of SUD treatment do not receive it. According to the 2015 NSDUH, approximately 21.7 million or 8.1 percent of Americans aged 12 years or older were identified as needing SUD treatment [1]. Yet in 2015, only 3.7 million Americans aged 12 years or older, or 14.0 percent of the United States population that needed treatment, received any substance use treatment for any kind of problem related to substance use. Among the 21.7 million individuals who needed substance use treatment, only 2.3 million people (10.8 percent) received specialty treatment [1]. According to the NSDUH, when substance use treatment was utilized, most individuals surveyed sought care in self-help groups (1.9 million) and outpatient rehabilitation programs (1.75 million). They less commonly obtained care in outpatient mental health centers, inpatient rehabilitation facilities, hospital-based inpatient programs, private doctor's offices, or emergency departments [2].

Deaths from Alcohol

Alcohol misuse and alcohol use disorders result in an estimated 88,000 deaths annually.

Alcohol misuse and alcohol use disorders result in an estimated 88,000 deaths annually [41], and excessive alcohol consumption is associated with adverse health and social consequences, including liver cirrhosis, certain cancers, fetal alcohol spectrum disorder, unintentional injuries, and violent behaviors [42]. Individuals with an alcohol use problem represent a heterogeneous population, which necessitates the use of personalized treatment approaches such as medication and counseling [43]. Medication-assisted treatment (MAT) incorporating pharmacotherapy and, ideally, psychosocial treatment, is an evidence-based treatment for alcohol use disorders; medications used include acamprosate, disulfiram, or naltrexone [44]. In 2015, 2.2 million people aged 12 years or older (0.8 percent of the population) received any type of past-year treatment for an alcohol use problem. Among these individuals, treatment was most commonly reported as occurring, non-exclusively, in self-help groups (57.5 percent), outpatient (33.5 percent) or inpatient (28.1 percent) rehabilitation facilities, outpatient mental health centers (26.6 percent), and inpatient hospitals (20.1 percent).[1] In 2015, approximately 1.4 million individuals reported receipt of specialty treatment in the past year for an alcohol use problem. This figure represented only 8.2 percent of the nearly 16.4 million individuals reported to need treatment for an alcohol use disorder. In 2015, only 12.9 percent and 7.8 percent of individuals who needed treatment and identified as non-Hispanic Black and non-Hispanic White, respectively, received it [2].

According to the NSDUH, in 2015, 22.4 percent and 17.4 percent of individuals receiving substance use treatment in the past year cited prescription opioid abuse or heroin use, respectively, as their reason for treatment [2]. Treatment for OUDs, whether related to heroin use or

[1] Percentages add to more than 100 percent because individuals may receive treatment in multiple settings.

prescription opioid misuse, is critical. In addition to the devastation caused by overdose, opioid use can have other serious consequences. For example, a longitudinal study examining the 27-year outcomes of heroin users found that heroin use predicted a 3-fold to 4-fold excess risk of premature death, even when substance abuse was not sustained [45]. In 2013, it is estimated that OUDs cost the United States more than $78 billion in health care, criminal justice, and lost productivity costs [46, 47]. Early and effective treatment is important.

Evidence-based treatment options for both prescription opioid and heroin use disorders include MAT with methadone, buprenorphine, or naltrexone, as well as behavioral therapies including cognitive behavioral therapy. Results for 18-month treatment outcomes from the Prescription Opioid Addiction Treatment Study found that, across ten study sites, nearly half of all study participants received MAT. Of those initiating treatment, 40 percent received buprenorphine, whereas only 6 percent received methadone treatment. Of prescription opioid users seeking treatment, 34 percent were engaged in psychosocial services and 40.9 percent reported participation in self-help groups [48].

Individuals with OUDs are not homogeneous. Different treatment approaches may be required, depending on the substance used and other individual characteristics. For example, one study found that individuals with a history of misusing prescription opioids were more likely to complete a substance use treatment program than were heroin users or individuals who engaged in combined opioid analgesic and heroin use [49]. Studies also suggest that individuals using prescription opioid analgesics may have better treatment outcomes with buprenorphine than individuals using heroin who receive similar treatment [49, 50]. Issues such as these indicate a need for individualized, patient-centered treatment.

Factors Influencing Participation in Treatment

Because so many individuals with SUDs do not obtain access to treatment, some exploration of factors that influence initiation and engagement in treatment is necessary.

Research shows that many factors may contribute to patients' initiation and engagement in treatment, including: (1) individual; (2) provider; (3) health plan; and (4) market and environmental factors. Figure 1 conceptualizes how multiple factors identified in the literature can affect this process.

We examine in greater detail below factors affecting treatment participation that have been identified or studied in the past 5 years.

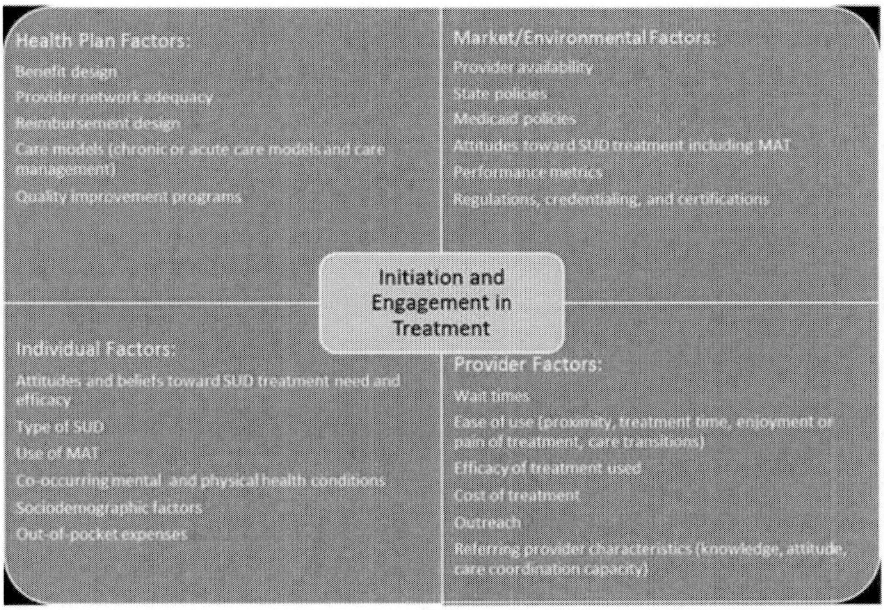

Figure 1. Theoretical Model to Explain Participation in SUD Treatment

Individual Factors

Research has shown that individual patient characteristics – including individual beliefs, sociodemographic characteristics, types of substance use and substance delivery modality, treatment experience, co-occurring mental illness, cognitive functioning, and patient activation – may influence treatment initiation and engagement.

Individual Beliefs

Individual factors, including beliefs, play a large role in an individual's decision about whether to seek treatment. The Surgeon General's Report on Alcohol, Drugs and Health stated that "stigma has created an added burden of shame that has made people with SUDs less likely to come forward and seek help" (p. v) [12]. Research shows that the vast majority of people do not seek treatment because of attitudinal or belief barriers (e.g., lack of perceived need, concerns about stigma, doubts about efficacy) [51]. For example, the 2015 NSDUH found that, of the group identified as needing specialty treatment, only 4.6 percent personally felt a need for treatment, and only 1.6 percent of the group needing treatment actually attempted to enter into services. Nearly 95.4 percent of all individuals identified as having a need for SUD treatment did not feel that treatment was necessary [2].

Sociodemographic Characteristics

Individual patient characteristics and sociodemographic factors such as sex, age, race/ethnicity, education, and insurance may influence decisions to initiate and engage in SUD treatment services. This topic has been studied extensively, and we briefly summarize the resulting findings below.

- Women may be less likely than men to engage in SUD treatment [7, 8, 9, 10].
- Studies are mixed regarding the effects of age on initiation and engagement, with some studies showing older age to be beneficial [7, 52, 53], others younger age [9], and some no effect of age [54].
- Studies examining racial or ethnic differences associated with treatment initiation and engagement also produce varied results, including poorer initiation among Black and Hispanic populations compared with White populations, and higher rates of initiation for Native American and White patients than for other racial and ethnic groups [7, 54]. Similarly, several studies show that, compared with the non-Hispanic White population, Black and

Hispanic populations may have lower rates of treatment engagement [7, 42, 55, 56]. Findings related to treatment continuation also identify somewhat similar results, depending on the substance used [55].

- Education level also influences treatment initiation and engagement for all racial and ethnic groups, with lower levels of formal educational attainment associated with failure to initiate and engage in treatment [54, 55].
- Having health insurance also is a predictor of engagement in substance use treatment. For example, individuals who were insured had 1.4 times the odds of receiving alcohol dependence treatment compared with their uninsured peers [9].

Co-Occurrence

A total of 8.1 million Americans aged 18 or older have both a past-year SUD and a mental disorder.

Substance Use and Treatment Experience

The type of substance use, the route of ingestion, and history of SUD treatment also may influence treatment initiation and engagement.

- Although the evidence is mixed and other factors may influence the results:
    - Compared with individuals abusing heroin, individuals who abuse prescription opioids are more likely to engage in treatment [57].
    - Individuals engaged in alcohol abuse may be more likely to engage in treatment compared with those who have heroin dependence [55].
    - Individuals with alcohol or cocaine use disorders may delay treatment longer than individuals with other types of SUDs [54].

- Substance users who injected opioids were less likely to complete treatment than those who did not inject [49], and individuals who never used opioids via a non-recommended route (e.g., injection or snorting) were more likely to continue in treatment and abstain from illicit opioid use in the final 3 weeks of a 12-week buprenorphine treatment program [52].
- A prior history of SUD treatment may be associated with delays in the initiation of treatment for current needs [52, 54].

Co-Occurring Mental Illness and SUD

Co-occurring mental health issues are not uncommon in the population of those with SUDs, with 8.1 million Americans aged 18 or older having both a past-year SUD and a mental disorder. This represents more than 40 percent of adults with an SUD and has repercussions for treatment, including initiation and engagement [2]. Studies examining the co-occurrence of psychiatric conditions and SUDs suggest that dual diagnosis may complicate treatment initiation and engagement [11, 52].

Treatment initiation in those with co-occurring mental illness may be complicated by several factors. A study by Brown and colleagues examined treatment initiation in a sample of adults with serious mental illness diagnoses including schizophrenia, schizoaffective disorder, major depression, and bipolar disorder [11]. Researchers defined treatment initiation as completing a pretreatment intake assessment, which required two in-person visits over the course of 2 weeks. The study results indicated that, unlike the general population, males with serious mental illness were 54 percent less likely than their female peers to initiate treatment. Brown et al. [11] also found that the specific serious mental illness diagnosis may influence initiation of treatment. Compared with participants with other serious mental illness diagnoses, study participants with schizophrenia spectrum diagnoses were less likely to initiate treatment (odds ratio = 0.44). Recent drug use also may be a factor in whether individuals with serious mental illness initiate treatment [11].

Predictors of engagement may differ from predictors of initiation for individuals with serious mental illness. Brown et al. [11] found that, although patient characteristics and mental illness diagnoses may influence initiation, these variables did not predict engagement in SUD treatment (defined as attending three or more treatment sessions). Rather, engagement was predicted by the presence of current drug dependence (compared with recent history of drug dependence), patients' positive feelings toward family members, and having a recent arrest. Dreifuss et al. [52] found that the co-occurrence of an SUD and major depression was associated with improved treatment engagement and outcomes for individuals receiving buprenorphine/naloxone treatment for prescription opioid dependence. An example of the interaction of individual factors is suggested by the fact that the presence of both a mental disorder and SUD may be more prevalent in women – a group that has lower overall rates of engagement in SUD treatment [58].

Co-Occurring SUD and Reduced Cognitive Functioning

Cognitive function may be another significant predictor of patient engagement. One study compared rates of therapy session attendance for patients with an SUD with or without cognitive impairment. Those with cognitive impairment were significantly less likely to attend all of their group therapy sessions compared with their peers without cognitive impairment [59].

Patient Activation

Although not specific to alcohol and SUDs, recent research has found that increased levels of patient activation are associated with greater likelihood of treatment initiation and engagement for a range of chronic health conditions [60, 61, 62]. Greene and Hibbard defined patient activation as "having the knowledge, skills, and confidence to manage one's own health." [61, 62]. In examining factors related to patient and family activation and accountable care organization (ACO) support for and investment in facilitation of such activation, Shortell et al. (p. 580) [63] found "high-level leadership commitment, goal-setting supported by adequate resources, extensive provider training, use of interdisciplinary care teams, and frequent monitoring and reporting on progress" to be associated with greater patient activation.

Provider Factors

Provider attitudes, access and availability, ease of use, referral source, and the type and efficacy of treatment provided affect an individual's initiation and engagement into SUD treatment.

Research published in the past 5 years confirms and elaborates on these five overarching themes.

Provider Attitudes

Just as stigma can negatively affect individuals' propensity to seek treatment, provider attitudes toward those with SUDs may interfere with willingness to work with that population [16].

Provider Access and Availability

Lack of provider availability is routinely cited as a barrier to patients engaging in treatment [17, 18, 19]. Provider-related financial concerns, such as issues related to third-party reimbursement [18] and including benefit limits imposed by payers [64], may reduce the number of providers willing to offer SUD treatment or restrict their ability to offer the full range of treatments that would otherwise be available. As the Mental Health Parity and Addiction Equity Act (MHPAEA) of 2008 is implemented, some of these impediments may be less pronounced as payers increasingly reimburse the provision of behavioral health care at parity with physical health care.

Provider Access

Lack of provider availability is routinely cited as a barrier to patients engaging in treatment, and provider-related financial concerns may reduce the number of providers willing to offer SUD treatment.

The number of providers available to offer treatment, including the number certified to provide MAT for OUDs, is one major factor that also influences access. Another is the number of certified providers who prescribe buprenorphine – one major MAT option for patients with opioid dependence. There has been a continued increase in the number of providers certified to prescribe buprenorphine in recent years, which subsequently has increased patients' access to treatment [18]. A national survey of physicians certified to prescribe buprenorphine [18] revealed that this treatment option is largely prescribed outside of specialty treatment settings, further expanding access to patients. In 2004, 76 percent of buprenorphine-certified physicians were actively providing buprenorphine treatment to opioid-dependent patients. In 2008, the rate grew to 86 percent. A related factor is the number of patients each buprenorphine prescriber may treat, which also affects the availability of treatment. In 2006, certified prescribers treated an average of 18.4 patients with buprenorphine/naloxone. In 2007, a new policy increased the number of patients that providers are eligible to treat, and the average number of patients treated per physician rose to 27.3 that year and to 39 patients per provider in 2008. A 2016 amendment to the federal regulation governing the number of patients and types of providers who may prescribe buprenorphine is expected to alleviate some of the impediments to provider availability and increase the average number of patients per prescriber as well as the number and type of certified prescribers [65].

Ease of Use

Ease of treatment use is important for initiation and engagement. One major barrier is length of time until an appointment or opening is available to a prospective patient. Longer lengths of time between an index appointment and a treatment initiation appointment have been associated with patients' failure to engage in treatment [7, 66]. Other research shows that decreased wait time is associated with improved retention [67]. Treatment in smaller facilities also may contribute to patients' continued engagement, possibly because of the more intimate and less stigmatizing nature of smaller settings [7].

Evidence-Based Treatments

Use of several evidence-based practices may be associated with increased engagement in SUD treatment, as suggested in recent research.

Referral Source

Referral source may be an important predictor of patients' initiation of SUD treatment. Research indicates that this may be influenced partially by system characteristics and partially by individual characteristics. Results from recent analysis of treatment episode data indicate that, in 2012, only 22.8 percent and 25.8 percent of all outpatient and intensive outpatient (IOP) admissions were self-referred, a larger percentage originated from the criminal justice system (49.4 percent and 43.9 percent), and the remainder were referrals from other sources. Short-term and long-term residential treatment also was largely non-self-referred: short-term (33.2 percent) and long-term (26.6 percent). In contrast, detoxification was most frequently self-referred: free standing residential (55.8 percent), hospital inpatient (74.2 percent), and ambulatory (50.0 percent) [68]. Given that detoxification and inpatient settings often are accessed in crisis, the referral source may be identified as the patient (rather than a source such as a health care provider) whereas residential, outpatient, and IOP settings are most easily and commonly accessed by referral. This suggests that lower rates of self-referral for outpatient treatment may be the best indicator of patient motivation, whereas referral sources for other forms of treatment may be more indicative of how the treatment system functions.

Other research finds connections between referral source and treatment that reveal links to both patient characteristics and system functioning. By analyzing admission delays to outpatient methadone treatment, Gryczynski et al. [54] found that individuals who were referred to treatment by a health care provider had lower odds of delayed treatment. In contrast, individuals who were self-referred or referred by the criminal justice system were more likely to experience a delay in initiating treatment. These findings suggest that system design and provider characteristics may be the predominant factor rather than patient motivation. In contrast, race or ethnicity also may play a role in conjunction with referral source. Acevedo et al. [7] found an interaction between referral source and the patient's race in relation to patient initiation in outpatient treatment. Among those receiving referrals from the criminal justice system, Native American individuals were more likely than White individuals to initiate treatment. Native American and Black patients also were more likely to initiate treatment than White patients when receiving a referral from a health care provider.

Use of Evidence-Based Treatments

Several evidence-based practices exist for the treatment of SUDs, with MAT, contingency management, motivational interviewing, cognitive behavioral therapy, and structured individual or family therapies serving as the most prominent treatments [69]. Use of these practices may be associated with increased engagement in SUD treatment. Recent research shows the following:

- Use of methadone or buprenorphine for treatment of OUDs positively influences treatment retention [70, 71].
- Contingency management, a psychosocial therapy offering positive reinforcement such as a voucher or prize for abstinence or treatment participation [72], is efficacious for maintaining abstinence from alcohol, cocaine, and opioids; for improving SUD treatment attendance; and for enhancing group cohesion and therapeutic alliance in early stages of group therapy [73, 74].
- Contingency management combined with other psychosocial therapy interventions such as motivational interviewing [72] or integrated MAT and mental health treatment [75] also is effective. Higher rates of service utilization have been seen for co-located mental health and methadone maintenance programs when contingency management in the form of a monetary reward also is provided [75]. One drawback of contingency management is the

potential for unsustainable treatment incentives because of funding restrictions.

- Motivational interviewing, which may be used to identify patients' personal barriers and readiness for behavior change relative to substance use [72], is another evidence-based practice that may support initiation and engagement. Motivational interviewing is used in many health care settings, including SUD treatment [76, 77], and it presents an alternative to directly inquiring about patients' inclination for behavior change. Instead, the intervention uses a four-step process that builds patient trust until the provider can facilitate a patient-developed commitment and action plan for change [76] This has been shown to help patients with alcohol use disorder reduce their drinking [78]. Motivational interviewing and treatment readiness group sessions, combined with monetary incentives for enrolling in substance use treatment and attending sessions, was associated with higher rates of enrollment in methadone maintenance treatment, re-engagement in treatment following a program discharge, and reporting a greater number of total treatment days and fewer episodes of heroin use [79].
- Receiving group therapy during the initial SUD treatment visit is another predictor of continued engagement [7].

Health Plan/Payer Factors

Health plan factors influence initiation and engagement in substance use treatment. For example, health plan policies related to reimbursement, benefit coverage, and types of credentialed providers included in a network all affect the development of an adequate network for plan beneficiaries and overall access to a care continuum. In addition, favorable cost-sharing or alternative payment arrangements such as pay for performance (P4P) and ACO-like models, as well as care management and quality improvement programs, may improve treatment initiation and engagement.

Benefit Design

Health plans historically have imposed coverage restrictions, including treatment limitations and financial requirements that limit the use of SUD treatment services. Limited health plan benefit arrays, including coverage of services or MAT medications, and caps on office visits may hinder substance use delivery care, ultimately impeding initiation and engagement [21, 22]. Although many of these barriers are changing with implementation of the MHPAEA, health plan policies can substantially affect provider access and ultimately patient engagement.

A national survey of private health plans examined how the plans managed specialty behavioral health treatment entry and continuing care in 2010. Prior authorization only was required for entry into outpatient SUD treatment by 4.7 percent of plans, whereas 73.4 percent required prior authorization for continuation of such treatment. Requirements for entry and continuation were more strenuous to obtain partial hospitalization, IOP services, or day treatment, with 94.9 percent requiring prior authorization for entry and 94.5 percent requiring authorization for continued treatment. Residential treatment was the most difficult to access, with 97.2 percent requiring authorization prior to entry and 95.2 percent for ongoing treatment. Prior authorization was based on medical necessity criteria, which were developed most frequently by either the plan or by the American Society of Addiction Medicine (ASAM). Most plans had formal standards to monitor wait times for routine and urgent care, but 30 percent lacked such standards for detoxification services [23]. Given the implementation of parity, it is expected that many of these impediments may have been alleviated.

A study by Grogan et al. (2016) examined state Medicaid plan coverage of the four ASAM levels of care: (1) outpatient services; (2) IOP services; (3) residential inpatient services; and (4) intensive inpatient services. Researchers used results of a survey and environmental scan conducted in 2013 and 2014 to determine that only 13 states and the District of Columbia covered all services included in the four levels of care, whereas 26 states and the District of Columbia provided coverage for at least one service in each of the four levels. The most common restriction in other states was residential treatment, with 21 states providing no residential treatment. Ten states did not cover IOP services. Only half of the states and the District of Columbia provided funding for recovery support services [24].

Coverage Restrictions

Health plan coverage restrictions, including treatment limitations and financial requirements that limit the use of SUD treatment services may hinder substance use delivery care, ultimately impeding initiation and engagement.

A 2014 HHS Substance Abuse and Mental Health Services Administration (SAMHSA) report on Medicaid financing of MAT found considerable differences between the states in the state Medicaid reimbursement and benefit limits for MAT. Common benefit design elements that influence access to MAT for both alcohol and OUDs include use of preferred drug status for selected drugs; requirements for prior authorization, step therapy, or psychosocial treatment; and quantity or lifetime limits [25].

Payment Models

Several studies have focused on the use of performance-based payment for SUD counselors. Among therapists treating adolescents for SUDs in a community-based treatment organization, the providers receiving US $50 for each month that they demonstrated competence in substance abuse treatment delivery and US $200 for each patient who received a specified number of treatment procedures and sessions were more likely than the control group to achieve the target rates of treatment procedures. Additionally, the adolescents in the study were more likely to initiate treatment, although there was no significant difference in patient remission status [66, 80]. Where counselors at a community drug treatment clinic could earn cash bonuses based on therapy attendance rates of individual clients as well as on the quarterly retention rates of their caseload, average therapy sessions attended during the first month of treatment increased from 4.6 sessions prior to the intervention to 5.5 sessions per client during the intervention. The 90-day client retention rate increased from 40 percent to 53 percent [81].

Some state substance use agencies have employed contracts with specialty substance use provider organizations that tie payment to performance across various metrics. One well-studied example is Delaware, which, in 2002, replaced traditional cost-reimbursement contracts with performance-based contracting. The state tracked capacity utilization and active patient participation in treatment to increase the number of people enrolling in and utilizing detoxification services in the state. From 2001 to 2006, the average occupancy rate increased at substance abuse facilities from 54 percent to 95 percent. Some of the more successful strategies to increase occupancy rates were extending hours of operation, enhancing the facility, providing salary incentives to clinicians and utilizing evidence-based therapies [82]. Subsequent studies found that rates of transition to continuing care treatment improved following implementation of performance-based contracting [81], and that waiting time declined by 13 days whereas treatment length of stay increased [83].

Payment Tied to Performance: Delaware Example

In 2002, Delaware replaced traditional cost-reimbursement contracts with performance-based contracting, and saw an average occupancy rate at substance abuse facilities increase from 54% to 95% from 2001 to 2006.

Studies also have examined the effect of using an ACO-like payment structure on SUD treatment. A qualitative study on the early effects of Medicare ACOs on behavioral health processes found that Medicare ACOs were minimally focused on improving processes to connect beneficiaries to SUD services; reasons cited included a perceived lack of referral resources and a lack of provider training within the organization [84]. Researchers also examined the effect of the Blue Cross Blue Shield of Massachusetts

Alternative Quality Contract (BCBSMA AQC) on SUD performance measures of identification, initiation, and engagement. The BCBSMA AQC incentivizes provider organizations to control the total cost of care while improving quality measures, but they did not include any measures related to SUD in their quality measure set to which incentives attached. The researchers found that the BCBSMA AQC payment structure had no impact on SUD performance measures [85].

A study that did not directly focus on substance use treatment identified some impediments to successful use of P4P, at least in certain contexts. A P4P compensation model that strongly incentivized primary care physician (PCP) quality outcomes resulted in PCP frustration at patient behavior, rather than stimulating greater support for patient self-management and activation. However, younger providers and those who were already more patient-centric were least likely to express this frustration [86]. This suggests that organizational strategies to support patient and family activation may be important to supplement the use of P4P [63], as well as strategies to support and educate providers.

Market, Contextual, and Environmental Factors

Market, contextual, and environmental factors either may contribute to or detract from access to SUD treatment. Examples of such factors that influence SUD treatment initiation and engagement may include geography, national policies, and state policies.

Geography and Regional Variation

Research has shown considerable geographic variation in treatment availability for SUD treatment generally, often locating treatment gaps in the South, Southwest, or Midwest. Results show gaps in availability of providers who accept Medicaid or who are licensed to provide buprenorphine for OUD [87], as well as limited public treatment services in areas with a high density of African-Americans [88]. A recent study examined geographic variation in OUD treatment need and admissions to opioid treatment programs (OTPs) accepting Medicaid. Of 1,151 of OTPs included in the study, only 65 percent accepted Medicaid. Most counties had no access to OUD treatment in OTPs for Medicaid enrollees, with the greatest gaps in coverage found in the Great Plains and parts of the Southeast. The highest rates of OUD, however, were found in counties in New England, Appalachia and some adjacent areas, and Western states. The analysis found clusters of counties with higher-than-average rates of OUD and lower-than-average treatment admissions to OTPs accepting Medicaid in the Southeast portion of the United States [87]. Fifty-three percent of counties in the United States do not have a physician with the waiver needed to prescribe buprenorphine [89].

National and State Policies

National policies can either restrict or improve individuals' access to health care services, especially regarding patients who are publicly insured. As the largest funder of SUD services [90, 91]. Medicaid plays an important role in facilitating access to specific treatment modalities. Medicaid policies that promote the use of MAT are critical to patients with OUD for their ability to engage in treatment [92]. Such policies include providing coverage for all forms of MAT, including naltrexone, buprenorphine, and methadone for OUD treatment [92]. An analysis of evolving state Medicaid policies between 2004 and 2013 found that many states implemented changes, including adding buprenorphine to preferred drug lists or adding MAT as a covered benefit, thereby promoting access to patient engagement in SUD treatment [92].

National waiver programs also can be instrumental in increasing access to SUD treatment providers. In 2002, the HHS Food and Drug Administration approved buprenorphine for prescription by providers who received a waiver from the Drug Enforcement Administration (DEA). Providers obtain this waiver after completing educational requirements specific to buprenorphine prescribing practices. Prior to the waiver, approximately 98.9 percent of United States counties were experiencing a shortage of opioid treatment providers [19]. By 2011, 9 years after the waiver program went into effect, the percentage of counties experiencing shortages decreased to 46.8 percent. In 2011, only 10.4 percent of the United States population resided in counties that were classified as having an opioid treatment shortage [19]. The 2016 statutory and regulatory changes regarding types of providers that may become waivered and the number of patients they can serve is anticipated to further improve access to treatment.

Single policy changes alone, however, may be insufficient to improve patient initiation and engagement in treatment. In 2007, Massachusetts implemented a statewide universal insurance law, incorporating SUD services as essential health benefits available to all state residents. An assessment of the law's effect on service uptake revealed that the rate of treatment initiation generally was similar to the rate observed prior to the law, and the need for SUD treatment remained relatively high [93]. Qualitative interviews with community-based SUD treatment organizations revealed that, although coverage had been expanded, patients experienced barriers to processing their insurance applications. Because the state no longer allowed citizens to benefit from acute or emergency service coverage under Medicaid's presumptive eligibility status, patients often could not access timely care for their SUD needs. Additionally, co-payments continued to represent a significant barrier to patients' treatment initiation and continued use of services [93].

In 2010, the Patient Protection and Affordable Care Act (Affordable Care Act) expanded both public and private insurance coverage, providing greater access to health care. With regard to SUD treatment, the Affordable Care Act eliminated lifetime caps on treatment services and restricted the annual caps that insurance plans can impose [94]. Reducing these insurance-related barriers to treatment may affect the number of individuals initiating and continuing to engage in SUD services, although lack of treatment resources in certain areas, as well as non-expansion of Medicaid in certain states, may continue to impede access to those services [95].

Additionally, the Affordable Care Act allows young adults aged 19-25 years to remain under their parents' insurance coverage. Initial assessments of the effect of the legislation on young adults' use of substance use services failed to reveal any significant change in treatment uptake [96]. However, given the relatively high rates of substance abuse for this age group [1], expanded coverage ultimately may promote increased uptake of treatment services.

Affordable Care Act

The 2010 Affordable Care Act eliminated lifetime caps on SUD treatment services and restricted the annual caps that insurance plans can impose.

Reducing these insurance-related barriers may affect the number of individuals initiating and continuing to engage in SUD services.

A study examining the direct effect of the MHPAEA on SUD treatment outcomes found that, after the first year of implementation, no significant change was observed in patient initiation or engagement [97]. However, the direct effects of this law on patient outcomes may be delayed as health plans adjust to and incorporate their new coverage requirements. Health plans also are still in the process of satisfying more recent regulatory requirements [98], which also will influence implementation.

Initiation and Engagement in Treatment

A basic requirement of successful SUD treatment is that the individual enter treatment and continue to participate long enough to benefit from what the treatment can offer. These steps of entry into treatment and treatment retention are commonly labeled as *initiation* and *engagement*. Without initiation and engagement, meaningful treatment does not occur.

Treatment initiation and engagement have been defined in different ways. *Treatment initiation* generally indicates that a patient has attended at least one treatment or assessment session after being identified as someone who needs treatment for alcohol or drug use disorder or following an admissions process [7, 11]. *Treatment engagement* implies continued treatment through additional visits, usually a specified number of encounters occurring within a set time period, which may vary depending on the study definition. *Engagement* also may be examined under the rubric of *retention* or *completion*. Presently, the most commonly used definitions are derived from the IET performance measure, which sets a minimum floor for initiation and engagement. We discuss the IET measure definitions in detail in the Methods section of this chapter, but the simple definitions are as follows:

- Initiation: the percentage of members who initiate treatment through an inpatient alcohol and other drug (AOD) admission, outpatient visit, IOP encounter, or partial hospitalization within 14 days of diagnosis [99].
- Engagement: the percentage of members with a diagnosis of AOD dependence who initiated treatment and had two or more additional services within 30 days of the initiation visit [99].

Initiation and Engagement Measures

Treatment Initiation

Indicates that a patient has attended at least one treatment or assessment session after being identified as someone who needs treatment for alcohol or drug use disorder or following an admissions process.

According to the National Quality Forum, performance measures "serve as a critically important foundation for initiatives to enhance healthcare value, make patient care safer, and achieve better outcomes" [100]. At this point, there are hundreds of performance measures, but the most prominent measure related to SUD treatment is the IET measure.

Treatment Engagement
Implies continued treatment through additional visits, usually a specified number of encounters occurring within a set time period.

The Healthcare Effectiveness Data and Information Set Measure of Initiation and Engagement

IET Measure Development and Adoption

The IET measure was developed by the Washington Circle group in partnership with SAMHSA and the National Committee for Quality Assurance (NCQA) and was designed to be calculated using administrative claims data [101, 102]. In 2004, NCQA included the IET measure in their Healthcare Effectiveness Data and Information Set (HEDIS) quality measures [101, 102]. The HEDIS is the most commonly used set of quality measures in the United States managed health care industry; over 75 percent of United States health plans use them to measure performance [103]. The IET measure is part of both the HEDIS Health Plan measures and the HEDIS Physician Plan measures [104]. In addition to use in the HEDIS measures, HHS uses the IET measure in many quality reporting programs, including the following:

- HHS Centers for Medicare & Medicaid Services (CMS) Adult Core Set of Health Care Quality Measures for Medicaid (Adult Core Set).
- Medicare and Medicaid Meaningful Use (MU) Electronic Health Records (EHR) for Eligible Professionals and the MU Stage 2 clinical quality measures, which now are part of the Merit-based Incentive Payment System (MIPS).
- CMS Medicare Physician Quality Reporting System, which is now part of the MIPS.
- Physician Feedback/Quality and Resource Use Reports.
- Physician Value-Based Payment Modifier.

- Health Insurance Marketplace Quality Initiatives Quality Rating System and Qualified Health Plan Enrollee Experience Survey.
- CMS Medicare Part C/Medicare Advantage (Part C Star Rating and/or Medicare Part C Display).
- CMS Medicare and Medicaid Financial Alignment Demonstrations.
- CMS Medicaid Health Homes.
- CMS Medicaid Innovative Accelerator Program.
- CMS Medicaid 1115 Waver on Institutions for Mental Disease (IMD).
- SAMHSA and CMS Behavioral Health Clinic (BHC) Quality Measures in use as part of the Section 223 Demonstration Program for Certified Community BHCs [104, 105, 106, 107, 108].

In addition, the IET measure is used by at least four state Medicaid programs to tie Medicaid reimbursements to health plan performance within state Medicaid ACOs. Those states are Maine, New Jersey, Vermont, and Oregon [109, 110, 111]. The IET measure was endorsed by the National Quality Forum in 2009 as measure number 0004 [104].

IET Measure Validity

Measure validity is critical if one is to draw conclusions from measure rates. Harris and colleagues have performed a series of studies to assess the validity of the IET measure, including assessing whether the codes used in calculation correspond to the receipt of substance use treatment [112, 113]. Harris et al. [114] and Garnick, Dunigan, and their colleagues also have examined the relationship of the measure to outcomes [115, 116, 117].

Studies of the relationship of IET codes to receipt of treatment originated in and used data from the Veterans Health Administration (VHA) National Patient Care Database. They assessed whether there was agreement between the code combinations and clinical progress notes regarding treatment. The first such study concluded that VHA SUD specialty facilities had high concordance with clinical progress notes (92 percent to 98 percent accuracy), whereas outside outpatient clinics had a concordance rate of 63 percent and non-SUD specialty inpatient units had a concordance rate of only 46 percent. The researchers concluded that, outside of SUD specialty clinics that were integrated into the VHA, patients may be counted as meeting the HEDIS measures even though they may not have received addiction treatment [112]. A follow-up study found the results in VHA SUD specialty clinics virtually unchanged (90 percent to 96 percent) accuracy. However, non-SUD outpatient and non-SUD inpatient clinics improved to 77 percent and 65 percent concordance with documentation of clinical progress notes, respectively [113].

Studies also show that IET rates correspond with some patient outcomes but not others. Harris and colleagues [114] found that individuals meeting the HEDIS engagement criterion had statistically significant improvements on the Addition Severity Index alcohol, drug, and legal composite scores, although the improvements were not clinically significant. Garnick and colleagues [116] found that engagement in publicly funded outpatient treatment services was associated with decreased risk of subsequent arrests. Dunigan and colleagues [117] examined the relationship between treatment engagement on employment using multiple outcomes of employment (i.e., any employment, wages, number of quarters employed, and hours worked).

Although they did not find a relationship between engagement and employment in the overall sample, they did find a relationship between engagement and employment and higher wages for those individuals with a history of criminal justice involvement. Similarly, Garnick et al. [115] found improved performance on multiple substance use outcomes among adolescents who engaged in treatment.

NCQA Quality Compass Data

Analysis of these data indicates that rates of initiation are higher than rates of engagement across all commercial, Medicaid, and Medicare plans.

Structure of the Measure, Including Non-inclusion of MAT

The process for calculating the IET measure rates is explained in detail in the Methods section of this chapter, as the initiation and engagement rates are dependent variables in quantitative analyses undertaken as part of this study. Performance measures, however, are updated often, most typically with minor revisions to codes used for calculation. Changes to the HEDIS version of the IET measure for 2018 included more substantive changes, such as one addressing the former non-inclusion of MAT in the calculation of receipt of substance use treatment as part of the measure numerator [118]. MAT is now a major part of SUD treatment for alcohol and OUDs, and the amendment addresses that fact, recognizing that initiation or engagement in treatment may include receipt of MAT. Other key changes for 2018 include the addition of services received by telehealth, stratification by age and diagnosis, and extension of the time measured to satisfy the engagement measure from 30 to 34 days. Many of these changes reflect the evolving nature of SUD treatment.

Health Plan Trends for the IET Measure

Since inclusion of IET in the HEDIS measures in 2004, considerable data have been generated that provide information on rates of initiation and engagement. Analysis of NCQA Quality Compass data indicates that rates of initiation are higher than rates of engagement across all commercial, Medicaid, and Medicare plans. Medicare initiation rates generally have been higher than either commercial or Medicaid rates and, for Medicare, Medicaid, and commercial insurance, rates for both measures tend to be lower for health maintenance organization (HMO) plans compared with preferred provider organization (PPO) plans.

Commercial HMO and PPO Plans

Figure 2 displays the initiation and engagement trends for commercial HMO and PPO plans from 2005 through 2014. Initiation rates are slightly higher for commercial PPO plans than for commercial HMO plans. However, rates for both have steadily decreased over the last decade. In 2005, 45.8 percent of commercial PPO plan members and 44.5 percent of commercial HMO plan members needing alcohol or drug services initiated treatment. In 2014, the percentages of commercial PPO and HMO plan members initiating treatment dropped nearly 10 percent for both categories to 36.1 percent and 34.7 percent, respectively. Rates of engagement, although much lower than rates of initiation, have remained stable across commercial PPO and HMO plans over the last decade. The mean rate of engagement for PPO plans is 15.4 percent, and the mean rate for HMO plans is 14.6 percent.

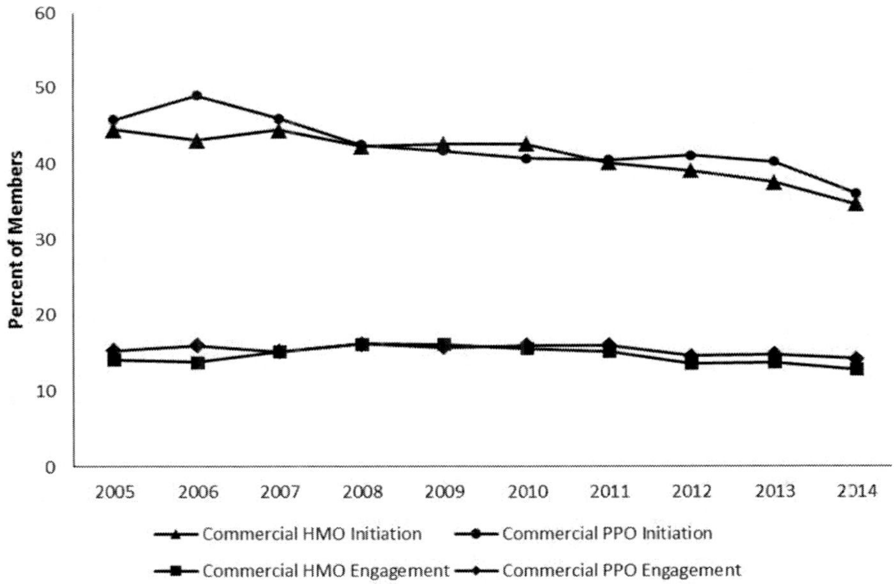

Source: Author summary of findings from NCQA Quality Compass data [119].

Figure 2. IET for Commercial HMO and PPO Plans, 2005-2014.

Medicaid HMO Plans

Figure 3 demonstrates the rates of initiation and engagement for Medicaid HMO plans from 2005 through 2014. Both initiation and engagement rates were highest in 2007 at 45.6 percent and 14.4 percent, respectively. Since then, rates for both measures have decreased. The last 3 measured years represent the lowest initiation rates recorded, as well as 3 consecutive years of lower-than-average engagement rates for Medicaid HMO plans.

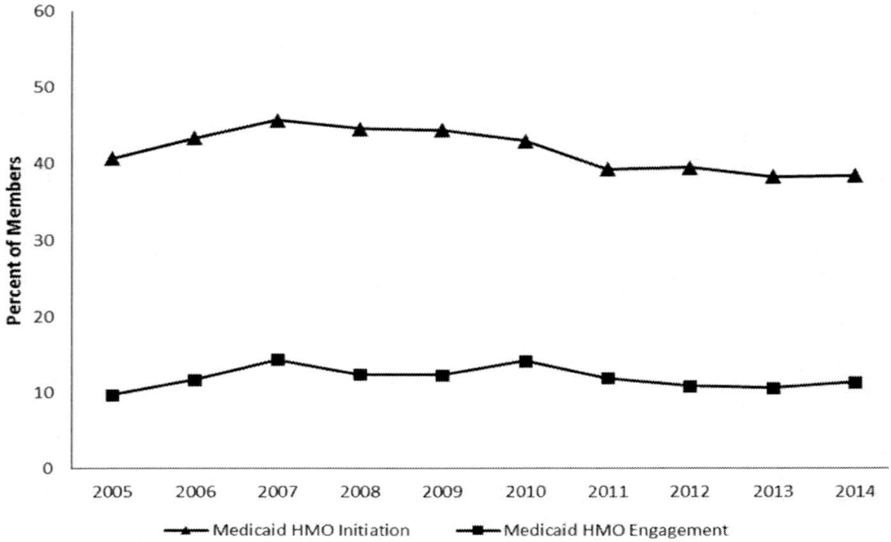

Source: Author summary of findings from NCQA Quality Compass data [119].

Figure 3. IET for Medicaid HMO Plans, 2005-2014.

Medicare HMO and PPO Plans

The average initiation rates for Medicare plans are higher than rates for plans under either commercial or Medicaid insurance (Figure 4). Across the last 10 years, Medicare HMO plans have averaged around a 43.4 percent initiation rate, compared with 41.6 percent in Medicaid and 41.1 percent in commercial HMO plans. The average initiation rate for Medicare PPO plans is even higher (48.6 percent), compared with the commercial PPO plan average (42.4 percent). As with Medicaid, Medicare plans experienced the highest rate of initiation in 2007, with 50.4 percent in HMO plans and 56.5 percent in PPO plans. While HMO plans have seen a steady decrease in initiation rates over time, initiation rates for Medicare PPO dropped in 2008 before spiking in 2009 and 2010; however, Medicare PPO rates have decreased substantially since 2010. In 2014, only 35.1 percent of those needing treatment initiated care in Medicare PPO plans and only 32.5 percent initiated care in Medicare HMO plans. Rates of engagement also decreased over time. Between 2006 and 2008, Medicare PPO engagement rates were higher than those associated with Medicare HMO plans. Since 2009, rates of engagement have remained similar and stable between both plan types. In 2014, 3.3 percent of those needing treatment engaged in care with a Medicare HMO plan, and percent engaged in services with a Medicare PPO plan.

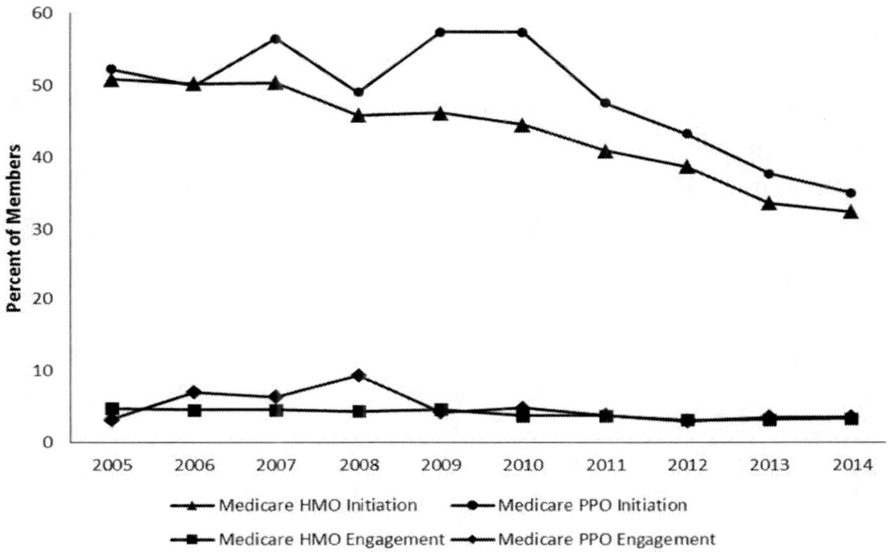

Source: Author summary of findings from NCQA Quality Compass data [119].

Figure 4. IET for Medicare HMO and PPO Plans, 2005-2014.

Interventions Designed to Improve Initiation and Engagement

Several best practices and intervention components for treating SUDs have been developed to address some of the barriers to initiation and engagement. One type of intervention that is discussed in the section above is the implementation of evidence-based clinical practices. Many of these practices have been shown to enhance treatment retention, and efforts to incorporate their implementation in facilities could be expected to increase initiation and engagement rates. There is not, however, complete consensus within the addiction specialist community as to which practices truly meet "best practice" standards [120].

In the section below, we discuss two other categories of interventions identified in the literature: (1) interventions that have been studied to address special populations; and (2) organizational interventions.

Interventions to Address Special Populations

Recent research has examined factors that are important in targeting SUD interventions for young adults, ethnic minorities, and individuals with co-occurring psychiatric illness. Many of these interventions focus on increasing the "fit" of the treatment with the targeted demographic as well as increasing availability and access to treatment through enhanced contact or coordination.

Young Adults

Young adults may respond to treatment differently than older individuals, and age-specific approaches may enhance initiation and engagement. Examples include whether they thrive and remain in treatment better when they are with individuals of similar age and whether they may be more likely to engage in treatment if a harm reduction model is employed.

Results are mixed on whether young adults do better when in treatment with people of similar ages. For example, younger adults face age-related challenges in engaging with other 12-step members [121]. Only 15 percent of Alcoholics Anonymous or Narcotics Anonymous 12-step members are younger than 30 years. Additionally, younger adults may find it difficult to identify other similarly aged individuals who are engaging in sobriety [121,122]. Thus, it may be challenging for younger adults seeking treatment to engage with the majority of members in these programs [122, 123]. Labbe et al. [123] examined 12-step meeting attendance among adults aged 18-25 years and found that the age composition of participants in meetings significantly moderated the effect of attendance on abstinence. The study results suggested that linking younger adults who were prone to non-adherence to meetings attended by similarly aged peers may improve treatment during the early phases of recovery. However, the results also suggested that continued attendance in meetings with peers of the same age group may be detrimental to encouraging long-term engagement. Research also shows that young adults prefer to reduce their intensity of substance use rather than to fully abstain from use [124].

Ethnic Minorities

Culturally relevant care also plays a major role in patient engagement. A qualitative study examining barriers and facilitators to SUD treatment engagement for American Indian and Alaska Native populations revealed that many providers employ a diverse array of health practices and culture-based interventions to deliver substance abuse treatment services [125]. SUD program directors and Single State Authority (SSA) representatives explained that incorporating traditional interventions created a supportive treatment environment for culturally diverse patients. Additionally, providers found that respecting cultural taboos, including not documenting healing practices, was useful to engaging Alaska Natives and American Indians in SUD treatment. To facilitate this culturally competent care delivery system, several providers and Single State Authorities reported conducting educational trainings with staff as a way to improve knowledge and use of the cultural interventions [125].

Co-Occurring Substance Use and Mental Disorders

Individuals with co-occurring substance use and mental disorders have a high-risk for treatment non-adherence and dropout [26, 126]. Specialized interventions may aid in increasing this population's initiation and continued engagement in care. For example, psychosocial interventions delivered through brief in-person sessions and follow-up calls with the patient, as well as through another family member, were shown to improve treatment adherence for individuals with bipolar disorder and a SUD [126].

Providers may need to pay special attention to younger adults with co-occurring SUDs and mental disorders. As previously stated, younger adults aged 18-25 years are at the highest risk for SUDs [1]. Recent research also suggests that individuals in this age group with serious mental illness are more likely to engage in substance abuse [92].

Integrated treatment may be a useful method for treating individuals with co-occurring needs and may encourage improved initiation and engagement. Integrated treatment focuses on providing health care services and monitoring two or more conditions, such as a mental health condition and SUD. Patients with integrated treatment often receive a combination of therapies, including psychotherapy and pharmacotherapy. Integrated treatment also may involve a team of providers including a PCP, psychotherapist, and social worker or case manager to help coordinate the patient's care [26]. In a recent review of empirical studies focused on treatment outcomes for individuals with co-occurring conditions [26], the authors found that case management is an important component in decreasing clients' needs for inpatient treatment and increasing their time in the community. Kelly and Daley [26] found that care models for patients with co-occurring conditions that emphasized the use of case managers who provided continuous support were associated with: (1) patients staying in the community longer; (2) decreased need for inpatient treatment; and (3) decreased drug use and psychosocial issues.

Organizational Interventions

In this section, we describe interventions implemented largely at the organizational level. First, we summarize the results of two large efforts at improving SUD treatment access and retention. These two initiatives were implemented across multiple states and providers to identify solutions to improve access to care and decrease "no-show" rates. Solutions often were individualized for each provider, but several overarching themes emerged. Themes from the results of these initiatives are summarized in Table 6. Second, we report on studies of enhanced outreach by providers and, third, on transformation to patient-centered service delivery. Fourth, we report on efforts underway that are not yet the subject of study but that reflect systematic approaches that may prove useful to improve SUD treatment access.

Multisite Interventions Aimed to Improve Access and Engagement

Between 2007 and 2010, 10 states participated in the Strengthening Treatment Access and Retention – State Initiative (STAR-SI) program conducted by SAMHSA [127]. Through this initiative, states developed innovative interventions to decrease the number of individuals who do not show up for SUD treatment in up to 15 of their local outpatient clinics. State-level results then were aggregated to determine which interventions were most effective in increasing linkage to care. As previously discussed, behavioral engagement strategies and reminder calls were efficacious in reducing no-show rates. Additionally, several outpatient clinics conducted organizational-level interventions to improve engagement [127].

Wait time was identified as a major barrier to appointment adherence. Among the 11 clinics reporting this barrier, the overall rate of patients who did not attend treatment that was attributed to wait time was 41.7 percent. Facilities implemented different organizational interventions to reduce their wait times, including offering walk-in appointments, double-booking appointments, and altering the way visits were scheduled. In one facility, the ability of providers to book their own appointments was replaced with a centralized appointment scheduling system. After implementing such interventions to reduce wait times, the overall no-show rate of patients that could be attributed to this factor was reduced by more than 20 percent [127].

Delays in the admissions process also were cited as a barrier to patients attending their appointments at STAT-SI facilities [127]. Treatment attrition during the admissions phase is a well-documented barrier to engaging patients in care. In a recent literature review, Loveland and Driscoll [128] found that attrition primarily occurs within the first 24-48 hours following patients' initial request for services and increases in likelihood with each day that a patient waits to begin treatment following their initial request.

Linking individuals to care on the same day as their initial service request was significantly associated with increased appointment adherence. Across the five studies they assessed, patients linked to treatment on the same day as their request were 2.5 times more likely to attend their treatment appointments, compared with individuals who waited 3-7 days for an appointment [128].

Within the STAR-SI study, some facilities opted to redesign their admissions process to reduce wait times between appointments. Most facilities altered their processes by reducing the number of steps required by patients before their first appointment, resulting in an over 20 percent reduction in no-show rates across all STAR-SI treatment centers [127]. Other approaches included increasing clinical capacity, which reduced no-show rates by 24.3 percent in six clinics [127]. Enhancing collaboration with SUD treatment referrers also helped decrease clinics' no-show rates. In some cases, collaboration was enhanced by asking the referrer to offer the client an incentive to attend treatment while, for patients referred through the criminal justice system, they advertised a penalty for not attending the visit. Finally, simply creating a more visually attractive and welcoming treatment environment through décor changes helped improve patients' comfort levels and decrease no-show rates by nearly 6 percent [127].

The Network for the Improvement of Addiction Treatment (NIATx) initiative presents another national effort to improve SUD treatment initiation and retention in local clinics. The NIATx model of process improvement for behavioral health encourages individual treatment facilities to first conduct an *agency walk-through* to better understand how patients interact with organizational elements of treatment including reception services, initial screening, assessment, admissions, and treatment planning processes [129]. A *change team* then is established to further identify barriers to treatment engagement in the current organizational processes and to design and implement interventions in a rapid-cycle testing environment. Continuous monitoring and evaluation of the interventions are conducted to assess improvements and determine where additional resources are needed [129].

Los Angeles County treatment facilities were included in a phased pilot study of the NIATx model between 2005 and 2008 [129]. Each of the SUD agencies identified its own improvement objectives on the basis of agency walk-throughs and a review of baseline patient engagement data. Change leaders implemented a variety of interventions to improve admissions processes and treatment retention and to reduce no-show rates. Interventions included increasing contact with prospective patients prior to admission, conducting same-day assessments to improve efficiency, and reducing the amount of paperwork completed for intake and assessment processes. Treatment facilities aiming to improve appointment adherence attached patient incentives to appointments, began providing physical appointment cards to patients, and conducted satisfaction surveys to continue engaging patients in treatment. Aggregate data suggested an 83 percent reduction in no-show rates related to assessment and intake barriers and a 39 percent increase in 30-day retention during phase one of the pilot study [129].

Phase two of the study included 12 SUD treatment facilities with similar improvement objectives. Facilities seeking to decrease the waiting time between patients' initial contact to their intake or assessment appointment developed various interventions [129]. For example, they merged preassessment phone interviews into a single interview that was conducted during the patient's first interaction with the facility. Other interventions included increasing assessors' appointment availability, offering walk-in assessment services, and sending case managers to prospective patients' homes to complete assessment paperwork. Following the interventions, the average wait time between appointments was 3.5 days – approximately 2.5 days shorter than the facilities' target [129].

SUD facilities that aimed to achieve overall decreases in their no-show rates for intake and assessment appointments relied on a combination of organizational and incentivized changes. Interventions included maintaining contact with waitlisted prospective patients through daily check-in calls, providing reminder calls the day before assessments, redesigning intake systems to include more assessment appointment times, adjusting appointment times to help clinicians complete paperwork in a timely manner, and providing bus tokens to incentivize patients to attend the appointments [129]. Another successful tactic involved assignment of patients by the primary counselor to a group schedule at intake and allowing counselors to complete new patient assessments at a later appointment. Aggregate data across all facilities with intake or assessment appointment goals demonstrated a 43.4 percent decrease in no-show rates [129].

Foci for Organizational Interventions

Interventions focus broadly on improving outreach, reducing wait times for both initial and subsequent appointments, using incentive programs, decreasing the complexity of the initial intake process, and improving the patient's experience.

Substance use treatment facilities seeking to improve 30-day retention in treatment adopted a practice of holding weekly meetings with patients during the first 4 weeks of treatment to assess patient satisfaction with the program and treatment plan [129]. Patients were asked to complete surveys regarding ways to further improve treatment. Facilities also adjusted their set meal, medication, and mail delivery times to better accommodate patients' schedules. The establishment of one-on-one welcome meetings between new patients and staff members from different departments within the treatment facility also promoted retention [129].

Several themes emerged among these initiatives as foci for organizational interventions (Table 6). Specifically, interventions were focused broadly on improving outreach, reducing wait times for both initial and subsequent appointments, using incentive programs, decreasing the complexity of the initial intake process, and improving the patient's experience.

Table 6. Themes for multisite improvement efforts to enhance initiation and engagement

Theme	Examples of Organizational Interventions
Enhanced outreach	• Making outreach calls with appointment reminders • Enhancing collaboration with the referral source • Increasing contact with patients prior to admission or with those on a waiting list • Providing physical appointment cards
Reduction of wait times for intake appointments or between appointments	• Increasing clinical capacity by hiring additional providers • Enhancing collaboration with referral source • Conducting same-day assessments or providing walk-in assessments • Centralizing appointment scheduling and increasing appointment availability • Having counselors assign group schedule at intake
Appointment incentives	• Advertising penalties for not attending appointments • Providing patient incentives for attending appointments, such as bus tokens
Decreasing complexity of intake processes	• Reducing paperwork for intake and admissions • Combining multiple preassessment interviews into 1 interview conducted during patient's initial contact • Having case managers make home visits to complete paperwork • Altering the length of appointments to allow providers to complete paperwork • Allowing providers to take more than 1 appointment to complete assessment paperwork
Improving patient experience	• Improving decor and environment to make it feel more welcoming • Using satisfaction surveys or meetings to assess patient satisfaction

Source: Author summary of reports of results of the STAR-SI [127] and NIATx [129] multisite studies.

Enhanced Outreach

Additional research examined the use of mobile phone strategies to decrease non-attendance rates. Patients who fail to attend appointments are more likely to drop out of treatment and experience poor outcomes [73] Meta-reviews of previous research suggest that appointment reminders sent through text messages to patients' mobile phones improve treatment attendance, compared with individuals receiving no reminders [130, 131, 132].

Text reminders represent an efficient intervention by health service providers to improve treatment initiation and adherence [130] and also may be a cost-effective alternative to traditional reminders through phone calls [132]. Mobile phone-based interventions also can be used to support patients' motivation for behavior change. Spohr et al. [133] found that regularly reminding patients of their short-term life goals resulted in higher likelihood of SUD treatment initiation and appointment adherence. Patients who opted not to receive text message reminders attended 56 percent fewer days of treatment. Additionally, phone calls reminding patients of next-day appointments have been useful in reducing the number of patients who do not arrive for intake and assessment appointments as well as in increasing treatment retention [73, 129].

Patient-Centered Service Delivery

Patient-centered care is a growing movement in health services, exemplified by the new emphasis on the creation of medical homes and integrated care models. This model, which encourages care coordination as well as shared decision-making and patient-centered care, is vastly different from more common models of addiction care. Specifically, individuals with alcohol use disorders traditionally have been offered standalone, group-based, 12-step programs [134]. Although these programs can be efficacious, they do not offer wraparound services or additional treatment options such as MAT, which may help engage some patients in care [134].

One aspect of providing patient-centered care is ensuring a high level of coordination between patients' providers. Patients who receive a greater level of coordinated care across their primary and specialty care providers, as demonstrated through jointly developed discharge plans and referral to local resources, remain in care longer than patients who do not receive such coordinated care [27]. Research suggests that the positive association between higher levels of continuity-of-care practices exists for both the general population of individuals seeking SUD treatment and for a subgroup of that population experiencing co-occurring psychiatric disorders [27].

Vermont

Vermont initiated the health home "hub and spoke" model in 2013 for individuals with OUDs and mental health conditions. This model uses regional opioid treatment providers as hubs to initiate treatment and incorporates a team of office-based opioid treatment providers to deliver ongoing support.

One model of patient-centered integrated care that is increasingly focused on patients with SUDs is Medicaid health homes. Although the results of these initiatives are not yet available, three states – Vermont, Rhode Island, and Maryland – have initiated Medicaid health homes for individuals with SUDs [135]. Medicaid health homes require six core services: comprehensive care management, care coordination, health promotion, comprehensive transitional care follow-up, individual and family support, and referral to community and social support resources.

Vermont initiated their health home "hub and spoke" model in July 2013 for individuals with OUDs and mental health conditions. This model uses regional opioid treatment providers as hubs to initiate treatment or provide care to complex patients, and it incorporates an enhanced team of office-based opioid treatment providers to deliver ongoing support for less complex patients [135].

Rhode Island also initiated Medicaid medical homes focused on individuals who receive or qualify to receive MAT [135] and have enhanced the services of their opioid treatment providers to offer the range of services required by a medical home. Finally, Maryland initiated their health homes in October 2013, for beneficiaries with OUDs and a co-occurring mental or physical condition and for individuals with serious and persistent mental illness. Their health homes are based in opioid treatment centers for individuals with SUDs and in either psychiatric rehabilitation programs or mobile treatment providers for individuals with severe and persistent mental illness [135].

Shared decision-making is another model of patient-centered care that can be useful for individuals with SUDs. When patients engage in shared decision-making with providers, their individual preferences, values, and needs are considered in treatment planning. Shared decision-making between providers and patients also ensures that patients have a better understanding of their medical conditions and are supported throughout the treatment process [76, 134, 136, 137, 138]. When patients are actively involved in health care and self-management decisions, they are more likely to engage in care and adhere to treatment [136]. Patient-centered care models can be used in addiction treatment to improve care coordination across primary and specialty care providers and to ensure that patients have access to all necessary resources to promote their full engagement and retention in care [139].

Promising practices also have been developed in areas that are not specific to SUD treatment. Care management models that incorporate such practices as frequent face-to-face contact, facilitated exchange of patient information among providers, and patient education and behavioral change techniques such as motivational interviewing, have been shown to decrease inpatient admissions among high-risk Medicaid enrollees with chronic conditions [140, 141].

Unstudied Systematic Approaches

Many systematic interventions are underway that have not been the subject of published studies. One such intervention is being promoted by the Healthcare Fraud Prevention Partnership (HFPP), which is a group of health plans, state and federal agencies, and others working to prevent fraud and waste associated with opioid prescribing. Although the focus is fraud and waste, they simultaneously are seeking ways to promote recovery from OUD. Priority actions that fall within this goal are: (1) promoting access to MAT; and (2) encouraging the use of data that can be used for activities such as identifying patients at risk of opioid misuse and OUD and providing intervention. The HFPP recommends use of cross-payer data to facilitate these goals. HFPP also seeks to identify and broadly disseminate effective methods for treating OUD. Although much of the HFPP effort relates to reducing inappropriate prescribing and misuse, the approaches being taken also can be instructive for promoting access to treatment. These include provider education regarding guidelines, continuing medical education credits, and a form of "academic detailing" that uses individual consultation. Patient education also plays a role, with HFPP members engaged in segmenting audiences to deliver information where it is needed and developing resources that fit the audience. A third focus, aimed at getting enrollees into MAT, includes approaches such as educating providers, use of technology such as the SAMHSA mobile app, promoting use of new pharmacological formulations such as implantable buprenorphine, promotion of Screening, Brief Intervention, and Referral to Treatment (SBIRT), and use of telehealth. HFPP also seeks to promote use of data to identify problems with opioid use and target corrective action. Some of the data systems available may be prior authorization systems, claims processing systems, and payer data warehouses. The HFPP is attempting to develop methods for its members to share such data but recognizes that constraints such as privacy may be a barrier. Similar barriers exist that often prevent health plans from accessing Prescription Drug Monitoring Program (PDMP) data. Drug utilization reviews, which presently may result in pharmacy lock-ins, are other potentially useful sources of information [142].

Another systematic approach was announced by the State of Oregon in 2017. The state plans to create a single point of shared responsibility for behavioral health needs for local communities through a regional governance model. The intention is to have all Oregonians served by a coordinated care model for behavioral health – essentially an expansion and modification of the Coordinated Care Organization model that has been in place since 2013 for Medicaid.

The model integrates care across systems, so all organizations in a community that are responsible for behavioral health (e.g., community mental health organizations, hospitals, law enforcement, schools, physical health care) will be part of a governance structure to ensure that local resources are used in the most effective way and that there is coordination of care [143].

Three health plans in California have developed their own approaches to dealing with opioid misuse. Partnership Health Plan of California, a Medicaid plan, approached prescriber education related to overprescribing through incremental formulary changes. These changes were accompanied by intensive education, including in-person regional meetings, webinars with remote facilitators, promoting local development of prescribing guidelines, academic detailing, technical assistance and support related to conversations with patients that encouraged use of outside authority as the rationale for unpopular changes, outlier review, and pharmacy lock-in. They also provided alternative benefits such as acupuncture and chiropractic care, even though these services are not part of the California State Medicaid plan. Blue Shield of California, a commercial plan, added formulary controls, provided utilization reports to prescribers meeting certain criteria, and offered provider outreach for prescribers with problematic prescribing. They also offered prescriber education, provision of alternative benefits, use of lock-in programs, opioid safety coalitions, and advocacy efforts related to drug disposal. Kaiser Permanente of Southern California launched a safe opioid prescribing initiative for all lines of business that had support from the plan's leadership. It used data to help providers see the scope of the overall problem as well as more specific problems, built collaboration teams, relied on peer pressure and support for clinicians, and invested in clinician education. They also offered formulary management, facilitated use of EHRs to incorporate decision support, endorsed and further developed emergency department and urgent care guidelines, enlisted pharmacists to ensure that they also had responsibility for improving opioid access, developed interspecialty support agreements, and provided patient education and support [144].

STUDY OBJECTIVES AND HYPOTHESES

The aim of this study is to expand on the literature concerning individual, provider, health plan, market, and environmental factors that influence initiation and engagement in SUD treatment services. Specifically, the research team examines how these factors affect health plan performance on the IET measures for both commercial and Medicaid health plans.

Acknowledging that the reporting parameters of the IET measures themselves may influence how health plans develop quality improvement initiatives targeting health plan benefits or how providers and beneficiaries interact with treatment services related to substance use, we aim to use stakeholder interviews to provide insight on measurement performance.

Thus, the study has two overarching objectives:

- Determine the models of care, quality improvement interventions, and best practices used by higher-performing health plans to improve initiation and subsequent engagement in SUD treatment.
- Describe the provider, beneficiary, and market factors that affect their ability to successfully initiate and engage beneficiaries in substance use treatment services.

On the basis of existing literature, the research team hypothesized that health plans that performed well on the IET measures would be highly integrated behavioral and physical health service models; they would reimburse for a variety of substance use treatment-related services including case management, routine outreach, peer supports, outpatient, inpatient, partial hospitalization, and residential treatment; they would have high network adequacy and provide financial incentives for providers; and they might be more likely to serve smaller markets in a community-oriented model rather than be plans with large beneficiary enrollment covering diverse populations and geographic areas.

METHODS

To determine the factors that contribute to health plan success in engaging plan members in SUD treatment and to identify a more effective strategy to measure engagement, we used a sequential, explanatory mixed methods study design where quantitative data were analyzed before qualitative data were collected to help explain results observed in the quantitative analyses. We initially conducted an environmental scan to provide background on: (1) the epidemiology of substance use, SUDs, and treatment; (2) factors associated with treatment initiation and engagement; (3) interventions designed to improve initiation and engagement; and (4) the development and use of the IET measure. The results of the scan informed both the quantitative and qualitative research that followed. The quantitative analyses relied on data from a large commercial health plan data set linked to geographic state-level market variables. Guided by the results of the quantitative analyses and the preparatory scan, we then undertook a series of qualitative case studies of health plans that were selected based on their performance on the IET measure and other critical characteristics (e.g., geographic distribution). This tripartite study design is depicted in Figure 5.

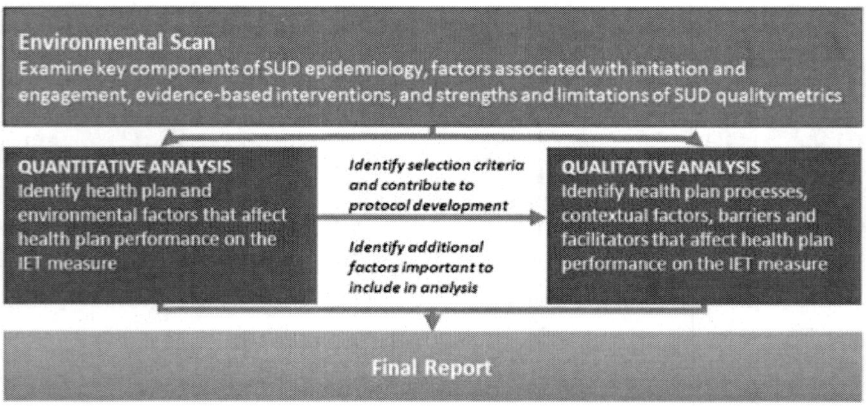

Figure 5. Tripartite Mixed Methods Study Design.

Quantitative Methods

Research Questions

The following research questions guided the quantitative analyses and include questions related to health plan and environmental factors regarding SUD treatment and OUD treatment.

Question 1: Do any of the following health plan factors affect initiation and/or engagement in alcohol or other SUD treatment?

a) Coverage of care continuum for SUD.
b) Out-of-pocket expenses for SUD treatment.
c) Reimbursement for outpatient and inpatient SUD treatment.
d) Percentage of population with an SUD.
e) Type of plan.
f) Plan beneficiary characteristics (age, sex, use of emergency department).
g) Number of beneficiaries.

Question 2: Do any of the following environmental factors affect a health plan's performance on initiation and/or engagement in alcohol or other SUD treatment?

a) Provider availability.
b) State demographic profile (race/ethnicity, poverty).
c) Prevalence of alcohol or SUDs.
d) Attitudes toward SUD treatment.
e) Policies to reduce opioid prescriptions for pain.

Question 3: Do any of the following health plan factors affect the initiation and/or engagement in SUD treatment for individuals with OUDs?

a) Coverage of care continuum for SUD.
b) Out-of-pocket expenses for MAT.

c) Reimbursement for outpatient and inpatient SUD treatment and for MAT.
d) Receipt of MAT for OUDs.
e) Percentage of beneficiaries with OUD.
f) Type of plan.
g) Plan beneficiary characteristics (age, sex, use of emergency department).
h) Number of beneficiaries.

Question 4: Do any of the following environmental factors affect a health plan's performance on initiation and/or engagement in SUD treatment for individuals with OUDs?

a) Availability of MAT providers.
b) State demographic profile (race/ethnicity, poverty).
c) Prevalence of OUDs.
d) State attitudes toward MAT as reflected in Medicaid coverage for all three medications for OUDs and SSA funding.
e) Policies to reduce opioid prescriptions for pain.

Data

For the quantitative analysis of factors associated with initiation and engagement among adults, we used the 2013-2014 Truven Health MarketScan® Commercial Claims and Encounters (CCAE) Research Database, linked to geographic information that provided state-level market characteristics. The MarketScan database is created from two sources: self-insured employers and regional health plans. For this study, we limited the data to those submitted by self-insured employers because this information includes all behavioral health claims.

We linked several state-level variables to the health plan data to provide information about the environmental context in which the health plan functions. We linked the data using the state where most plan beneficiaries live. Our primary goal with these variables was to assess the following environmental characteristics: (1) provider availability; (2)

underlying prevalence of alcohol and other substance disorders; (3) attitudes toward SUD treatment; and (4) state demographic characteristics. We considered several publicly available data sources to provide the environmental variables. The databases we selected to incorporate these characteristics are included in our description of covariates in Table 9.

Study Population

The unit of analysis for this study is the employer health plan. Table 7 describes the number of employer health plans with more than 10, 20, 30, and 50 beneficiaries that met the denominator criteria for the IET measure. It also includes the number that met those denominator criteria if restricted to beneficiaries with OUDs. Because comparatively few plans had sufficient eligible beneficiaries with OUDs to allow meaningful analysis, we implemented a requirement for 20 or more cases (as is done in some CMS reporting practices) and used data from both 2013 and 2014. This allowed us to include 321 health plans in our larger analysis of the rates for SUD treatment, with a mean of 50,585 beneficiaries, and 82 plans for the analysis of the rates for OUD treatment, with a mean of 92,521 beneficiaries. Because the IET measure requires that an Index Episode Start Date (IESD) be established with a 60 day "clean period" immediately preceding the IESD, we also used data from the end of 2012 to assure a clean period for those with episodes beginning early in 2013. More information on the IESD and related clean period is provided in the methods summary of outcome variables.

Table 7. Number of employer health plans with more than 10, 20, 30, and 50 beneficiaries meeting the denominator criteria for the IET measure, overall and limited to those with OUDs, 2013-2014

Measure	More than 10 Beneficiaries	More than 20 Beneficiaries	More than 30 Beneficiaries	More than 50 Beneficiaries
Overall				
Denominator	603	321	209	115
Limited to OUDs				
Denominator	178	82	43	16

Source: Truven Health MarketScan CCAE Research Database.

Beneficiary Population

The beneficiary population for the health plans studied included all adults (aged 18 years and older) with an alcohol or other drug (AOD) diagnosis who were enrollees in the employer health plans that contributed data to the 2013-2014 MarketScan CCAE data. As discussed in greater detail below regarding the outcome variables, an IESD was established for that group; any adults who did not have a 60 day "clean period" prior to the IESD were excluded from the beneficiary population used for rate calculation. For the analyses that focused only on those with OUD disorders, the beneficiary population was further reduced to include only that subset of the larger group.

Outcome Variables

Four outcome variables were included in these analyses (Table 8). The outcome variables were derived from the commonly used measure of IET, discussed in greater detail below.

Table 8. Outcome variables

Variable Name	Data Source	Description
Initiation SUD	MarketScan CCAE Database	As specified in the IET measure for AOD dependence treatment initiation[a]
Engagement SUD	MarketScan CCAE Database	As specified in the IET measure for AOD dependence treatment engagement
Initiation OUD	MarketScan CCAE Database	Amended the specifications from the IET measure for AOD dependence treatment initiation so that it only included the services with OUD diagnoses for identification
Engagement OUD	MarketScan CCAE Database	Amended the specifications from the IET measure for AOD dependence treatment engagement so that it only included the services with OUD diagnoses for identification

[a] NCQA. HEDIS & Quality Measurement, HEDIS Measures, HEDIS 2014, Volume 2: Technical Specifications. http://www.ncqa.org/hedis-quality-measurement/hedis-measures/hedis-2014.

The initiation rate is the Initiation Numerator divided by the IET Denominator.[a]

IET Denominator

- Identify all members who were aged 18 years or older as of December 31 of the measurement year.
- For those members, identify the Index Episode (this establishes the IESD, or the date from which measurement occurs):
  - o Identify those who, during the Intake Period (on or between January 1 to November 15 of the measurement year), had at least 1 OP, IOP, PH, detoxification, or ED visit with an AOD diagnosis, or an acute or non-acute IP discharge with an AOD diagnosis or AOD procedure code with the discharge date during the Intake Period. Select the earliest of these visits during the Intake Period; this is the IESD.
    - ▪ If the Index Episode is an IP event, the IESD is the date of discharge.
    - ▪ If the Index Episode is an OP, IOP, PH, detoxification, or ED visit not resulting in an IP stay, the IESD is the date of service.
    - ▪ If the Index Episode is an ED visit that results in an IP stay, the IP stay is the Index Episode and the IP discharge is the IESD.
    - ▪ For direct transfers, the IESD is the discharge date from the last admission.
- Test for NDH (this establishes that there is a 60 day "clean period" with no visits or encounters related to AOD in the period before the Index Date):
  - o Exclude members with a claim or encounter with an AOD diagnosis during the 60 days before the IESD.
    - ▪ For an IP IESD, use the admission date to determine the 60-day NDH period.
    - ▪ For an ED visit resulting in an IP stay, use the ED date of service to determine the 60-day NDH period.
    - ▪ For direct transfers, use the first admission to determine the NDH period.
- Include those who were continuously enrolled for the 60 days prior to the IESD through 44 days after the IESD (105 today days) with no gap.
- Exclude those with an IP stay with a discharge date after December 1 of the measurement year.

Initiation Numerator

- Identify those in the denominator. From those, include the following as initiation compliant:
  - o If the Index Episode was an IP discharge, the person initiated.
  - o If the Index Episode was an OP, IOP, PH, detoxification, or ED visit, initiation occurs if there was an IP admission, another OP, IOP, or PH visit (but not detoxification) with an AOD diagnosis, on the IESD or in the 13 days after the IESD (14 days total).
    - ▪ If the IESD and initiation visit are on the same day, they must be with different providers.

[a] See https://www.qualitymeasures.ahrq.gov/summaries/summary/49778/engagement-of-alcohol- and-other-drug-aod-treatment-percentage-of-members-who-initiated-treatment-and-who-had- two-or-more-additional-services-with-a-diagnosis-of-aod-within-30-days-of-the-initiation-visit.

Access the NCQA website or Medicaid Adult Core Set website for related value sets.

Figure 6. Initiation Rate Calculation Process.

The IET quality measure contains separate rates for initiation and engagement, with engagement measured among those who have initiated treatment. The IET quality measure defines initiation and engagement as follows:

- Initiation: the percentage of members who initiate treatment through an inpatient AOD admission, outpatient visit, IOP encounter, or partial hospitalization within 14 days of diagnosis [99].
- Engagement: the percentage of members with a diagnosis of AOD dependence who initiated treatment and had two or more additional services with an AOD diagnosis within 30 days of the initiation visit [99].

In these analyses, each rate was used twice – first, to measure initiation and engagement in AOD dependence treatment and second, to measure initiation and engagement in OUD treatment for those health plan members with OUD diagnoses. Appendix B provides the list of diagnoses included for OUD and other SUD analyses.

The IET specifications used to measure initiation and engagement in this study are those that are published by NCQA as HEDIS measures, which may be obtained through the NCQA website [103]. The NCQA specifications are similar to those used for the Medicaid Adult Core Set, although the Adult Core Set only applies to Medicaid enrollees and there are differences in the age ranges covered. The 2016 CMS Medicaid Adult Core Set is publicly available on the CMS website [105]. The value sets that include the codes needed to calculate the measure also are located on the CMS website [145], or they may be acquired with the NCQA specification.

Copyright considerations preclude including the NCQA specifications or the NCQA and Adult Core Set value sets as an appendix to this document. Figure 6 and Figure 7, however, depict the process of rate calculation for the IET measure.

The engagement rate is the Engagement Numerator divided by the IET Denominator.[a]
IET Denominator: Same as Denominator in Figure 6.
Engagement Numerator

- Identify those who were initiation compliant (see Figure 6). From those, include the following as engagement compliant:
  - Engagement occurs if there were 2 or more IP admissions, OP IOP, or PH visits with an AOD diagnosis, beginning the day after the initiation encounter through 29 days after the initiation (29 total days).
    - If the 2 visits are on the same day, they must be with different providers to count as 2 visits.
    - If initiation was via IP admission, the 29-day period begins the day after discharge.

[a.] See https://www.qualitymeasures.ahrq.gov/summaries/summary/49778/engagement-of- alcohol-and-other-drug-aod-treatment-percentage-of-members-who-initiated-treatment- and-who-had-two-or-more-additional-services-with-a-diagnosis-of-aod-within-30-days-of- the-initiation-visit. Access the NCQA website or Medicaid Adult Core Set website for related value sets.

Figure 7. Engagement Rate Calculation Process.

Covariates

We included covariates in our quantitative analyses that addressed five types of potential influences that were based on the results of our environmental scan, in which we examined the literature on factors that may promote or inhibit initiation and engagement in SUD treatment. These included: (1) health plan structure; (2) reimbursement factors; (3) benefit design; (4) plan beneficiary characteristics; and (5) state-level market and environmental characteristics. Table 9 describes in detail the variables within each category.

Table 9. Covariates

Variable Name	Data Source	Description
Health Plan Structure		
Plan type	MarketScan CCAE Database	Categorical variable indicating health plan structure as: (1) PPO; (2) HMO or capitated; or (3) high deductible health plan.[a] For regressions, PPO was the reference group.
Reimbursement Factors		
MAT OOP	MarketScan CCAE Database	Median OOP cost per user for MAT medications for OUDs (paid by enrollee).[b]

Table 9. (Continued)

Variable Name	Data Source	Description
Reimbursement Factors		
Outpatient OOP	MarketScan CCAE Database	Median OOP cost per user for SUD outpatient services, including IOP treatment and partial hospitalization services (paid by enrollee).
Inpatient OOP	MarketScan CCAE Database	Median OOP cost per user for SUD inpatient and residential services within health plan (paid by enrollee).
MAT reimbursement	MarketScan CCAE Database	Median reimbursement per user to pharmacy for MAT medications for OUDs (paid by enrollee and insurer).[b]
Outpatient reimbursement	MarketScan CCAE Database	Median reimbursement per user to outpatient providers, including for IOP and partial hospitalization services (paid by insurer).
Inpatient reimbursement	MarketScan CCAE Database	Median reimbursement per user to inpatient and residential providers for SUD services (paid by insurer).
Benefit Design		
MAT use	MarketScan CCAE Database	Categorical variable indicating percentage of beneficiaries with OUD who received: (1) no MAT; (2) buprenorphine/naloxone, extended-release naltrexone, or methadone (if coded in the claims) for 14 days or less (assumed to be for detox); or (3) buprenorphine/naloxone, XR naltrexone, or methadone for more than 14 days (assumed to be for maintenance).[b]
Residential	MarketScan CCAE Database	Boolean indicator that a health plan covers residential SUD services as evidenced by having at least one or more claims for each category of service.
Intensive outpatient (IOP) or partial hospitalization services	MarketScan CCAE Database	Benefit availability of IOP or partial hospitalization SUD services defined as the number of IOP or partial hospitalization services per plan beneficiary.
Outpatient services	MarketScan CCAE Database	Benefit availability of outpatient SUD services defined as the number of outpatient SUD services per plan beneficiary.
Health Plan Beneficiary Characteristics		
SUD beneficiaries	MarketScan CCAE Database	Percentage of beneficiaries/member-years within health plan with either an identified SUD diagnosis on a medical claim (non-laboratory and non-radiology) or receipt of MAT prescription. See Appendix C for the algorithm used to ascertain SUD beneficiaries.[c]

Variable Name	Data Source	Description
Health Plan Beneficiary Characteristics		
OUD beneficiaries	MarketScan CCAE Database	Percentage of beneficiaries/member-years within health plan with either an identified OUD diagnosis on a medical claim (non-laboratory and non-radiology) or receipt of a MAT prescription.[b]
Ages 18-44 years	MarketScan CCAE Database	Percentage of beneficiaries in a plan who were within the age group of 18-44 years.
Female	MarketScan CCAE Database	Percentage of beneficiaries in a plan who were female.
ED use	MarketScan CCAE Database	Percentage of beneficiaries in a plan with an SUD (or OUD) who had: (1) 0 treat-and-release ED visits with any diagnosis; (2) 1 treat-and-release ED visit with any diagnosis; or (3) 2+ treat-and-release ED visits with any diagnosis.
State-Level Market and Environmental Characteristics[d]		
SUD prevalence	2013-2014 NSDUH [146]	State-level data on the prevalence of alcohol and illicit drug abuse and dependence. Because health plans may have members in multiple states, the variable was the mean prevalence of the adult population with past-year dependence on or abuse of illicit drugs or alcohol in states where health plan members reside.[c]
Opioid prescriptions	2012 CDC infographic: [147] Number of opioid pain prescriptions per 100 people by state	The infographic provided the number of opioid pain prescriptions by state per 100 adults. Because health plans may have members in multiple states, the variable was the mean number of opioid pain prescriptions per 100 adults in states where health plan members reside.[b]
SUD capacity	2013 N-SSATS [148]	The data provided the number of adults receiving treatment in SUD treatment facilities by state per 100,000 adults. Because health plans may have members in multiple states, the variable was the mean number of individuals receiving SUD specialty treatment per 100,000 adults in states where health plan members reside.[c]
OTP capacity	2013 N-SSATS [148] for methadone number	The data provided the number of OTP spaces available for methadone treatment by state per 100,000 adults. Because health plans may have members in multiple states, the variable was the mean number of OTP spaces available per 100,000 adults in states where health plan members reside.[b]

Table 9. (Continued)

Variable Name	Data Source	Description
State-Level Market and Environmental Characteristics[d]		
Buprenorphine prescribers	SAMHSA Buprenorphine Physician Locator [149] US Census data for population aged 18 and over [150]	The buprenorphine locator identified the number of buprenorphine prescribers per state. The census data provided population aged 18 or older by state. Because health plans may have members in multiple states, the variable was the mean number of prescribers per 100,000 adults in states where health plan members reside.[b]
Six MAT medications	Medicaid Coverage and Financing of Medications to Treat Alcohol and OUDs (SAMHSA publication) [25]	The publication provided information on state Medicaid coverage of MAT medications as of 2011-2012. The variable was the percentage of health plan members who live in a state that covers all 6 medications for alcohol and OUDs: disulfiram, acamprosate, methadone, buprenorphine/naloxone, naltrexone, and extended-release naltrexone.[c]
Three MAT medications	Medicaid Coverage and Financing of Medications to Treat Alcohol and OUDs (SAMHSA publication) [25]	The publication provided information on state Medicaid coverage of MAT medications as of 2011-2012. The variable was the percentage of health plan members who live in a state that covers all 3 medications for OUDs: methadone, buprenorphine/naloxone, and naltrexone or extended-release naltrexone.[b]
Non-Hispanic White	US Census data [151]	The census data provided the percentage of the population in each state who identified as non-minority (i.e., non-Hispanic White) versus minority. Because health plans may have members in multiple states, the variable was the mean percentage of the adult population that was non-Hispanic White in states where health plan members reside.
Poverty	US Census data [152]	The census data provided the percentage of the population in each state who were below the 100 percent Federal Poverty Threshold. Because health plans may have members in multiple states, the variable was the mean percentage of the adult population that was below the poverty threshold in states where health plan members reside.
Private insurance	US Census data [153]	The census data provided the percentage of the population in each state who have private, commercial insurance.

Variable Name	Data Source	Description
State-Level Market and Environmental Characteristics[d]		
		Because health plans may have members in multiple states, the variable was the mean percentage of the adult population that has private insurance in states where health plan members reside.
PDMP	2015 Annual Review of PDMPs by the National Alliance for Model State Drug Laws [154]	State-level data that describe which states require prescribers and/or dispensers to access the PDMP in certain circumstances. The variable was the percentage of health plan members who live in one of the 24 states that required prescribers or dispensers to access the PDMP in certain circumstances in 2014.
Single state authority (SSA) spending	SAMHSA Publication: Funding and Characteristics of Single State Agencies for Substance Abuse Services and State Mental Health Agencies, 2013 [155]	The data provide the total amount of SSA spending on SUDs by state per 100,000 adult population. Because health plans may have members in multiple states, the variable was the mean amount of SSA spending per 1,000 adults in states where health plan members reside.

[a] Although plan type is self-reported, we verified that the self-report has a high match rate with health plan booklets.

[b] This variable was used only in the second analyses related to OUDs.

[c] This variable was used only in the first analyses and not the analyses related to OUDs.

[d] In order to calculate the environmental and market characteristics that use state-specific data, each health plan member was attributed to a specific state of residence and each state characteristic was assigned to each beneficiary according to his or her state of residence. For discrete variables, we use the percentage of individuals who resided in states with that characteristic. For continuous variables, we calculated the mean for the health plan, based on the mean of the individuals that make up the plan. For example, if beneficiaries 1-10 in health plan A lived in state X, then they were assigned the characteristics from state X. If beneficiaries 11-15 lived in state Y, then they were assigned the characteristics from state Y. The health plan variables were the mean of the beneficiaries' market characteristics.

Analytic Approach

We calculated descriptive statistics separately, focusing on SUDs and OUDs. We examined characteristics of the health plan cohorts used for the overall SUD analysis and the more specific OUD analysis. We calculated mean initiation and engagement rates on the basis of health plan characteristics. For continuous variables, we calculated separate mean initiation and engagement rates for health plans that performed at or above the health plan mean and those that performed below the health plan mean.

We examined plan characteristics by performance. For the SUD initiation and engagement measures, we divided the plans into tertiles on the basis of performance. For the OUD initiation and engagement measures, we divided the plans into those performing above the median (i.e., high performing plans) and those performing below the median (i.e., low performing plans). We then completed four multivariate regressions using general linear model analysis, examining the relationship between the covariates described above and the initiation and engagement measure outcomes. The separate regressions addressed initiation and engagement measure outcomes for SUD treatment and for OUD treatment alone.

Qualitative Methods

Research Questions

Three primary research questions guided the qualitative analyses to help us determine how successful health plans improve enrollee initiation and engagement in SUD and OUD treatment.

Question 1: Which types of health plan characteristics and strategies are demonstrated by plans with higher performance or greater improvement in IET in SUD and OUD treatment?

Question 2: What other factors (e.g., patient, setting, provider, state, and local market characteristics) do health plans identify as affecting rates of initiation and engagement in SUD and OUD treatment?

Question 3: What do health plan representatives believe are significant barriers and facilitators to initiating and engaging beneficiaries in SUD treatment?

Protocol and Discussion Guide Development

To guide the health plan interviews, we developed a combined site visit protocol and discussion guide document. The protocol component of this document contains logistical information to prepare the research team for specific site visits. Protocol elements included a list of all interviewees and their health plan division, position titles, and contact information. The document also included a site visit agenda, which indicated how interviewees were grouped and the key focus of their specific interview session. The final pages of the protocol included useful background information for the research team conducting the site visit. This background provided an overview of the health plan, relevant news articles related to the plan, and the plan's marketplace activity. This section also included information from documents sent by the plan prior to the site visit. The background information is described in further detail under Preliminary Data Collection.

We developed the discussion guide component of the document to identify facilitators and barriers to initiating or engaging health plan beneficiaries in SUD treatment. Major topic areas included health plan descriptive characteristics such as governance structure, benefit design, care models, reimbursement procedures and rates, network adequacy, and quality improvement methods; community and market characteristics such as state and Medicaid policies; patient factors such as use of MAT and attitudes and beliefs toward SUD treatment; provider characteristics such as billing proficiency, stigma toward SUD, outreach efforts, and use of evidence-based practices; and facilitators and barriers to initiation and engagement in treatment.

The guide includes semi-structured, open-ended interview questions to promote discussion and elicit the full range of potential responses from interviewees. Each semi-structured interview question includes a short list of optional probes to facilitate clarification and expand on the main question. Interview questions were designed to be flexible enough to allow the interviewer to stray from the guide if participant answers raise themes that the site visit lead deemed of value to the research questions. Following the first site visit, the research team made minor revisions to a few questions to promote a more natural language flow throughout the interview questions. The site visit protocol and discussion guide is attached as Appendix D.

Site Selection

We selected health plans for site visits on the basis of their performance across various behavioral health measures reported in NCQA data. Health plan performance was based on the most recent data available, which differed for commercial and Medicaid plans. The study analyzed NQCA Quality Compass data for commercial plan performance between January 1, 2015, and December 31, 2015, and for Medicaid plan performance between January 1, 2014, and December 31, 2014. The NCQA HEDIS measure data captures at least 75 percent of health plans in the United States.

Health plans initially were assessed on the basis of their HEDIS IET measure performance. The research team stratified the 396 commercial plans to identify plans performing in the 95th percentile on either the initiation (n=20) or engagement (n=20) measures. Among the 40 commercial plans identified, 17 were selected for extremely high performance either on one of the two measures or on both. Only seven plans performed in the 95th percentile on both measures. We repeated the stratification process on the 182 Medicaid plans to identify top performers on initiation (n=10) and engagement (n=10) measures. A total of ten Medicaid plans were selected for high performance, although only four Medicaid plans were identified as top performers on both measures.

Health Plan Selection

We selected health plans for site visits on the basis of their performance across various behavioral health measures reported in NCQA data.

Top-performing commercial and Medicaid plans also were assessed for their performance across several other HEDIS behavioral health measures of interest, including: (1) antidepressant medication management for the effective acute and continuation phases of treatment; (2) 7-day and 30-day follow-up after hospitalization for mental illness; and (3) mental health utilization of any IOP or partial hospitalization, or inpatient services.

Additionally, we assessed two composite measures from the Consumer Assessment of Healthcare Providers and Systems (CAHPS) measurement set, including customer service and getting needed care.

We prioritized for site visit selection any commercial and Medicaid plans identified as performing in the top 5 percent for both components of the IET. We also prioritized for site visit selection health plans that performed well on only one component of the IET and also performed well across the other behavioral health measures. High performance on the antidepressant medication management acute phase and 7-day follow-up after hospitalization for mental illness measures was favored over high performance on the other behavioral health measures because of the immediacy of measured outreach. To ensure that the health plans selected for site visits reflected geographic and socioeconomic diversity, as well as differences in state health policy, the research team also considered the state in which the health plan was located – including whether it was operating in a Medicaid expansion state – and its total enrollment size. We identified for secondary outreach an additional group of commercial and Medicaid plans with slightly lower IET, behavioral health measure performance, or both, should the prioritized plans not agree to participate in the site visits. However, this group of plans was not outreached because the researchers were able to schedule visits with the prioritized plans.

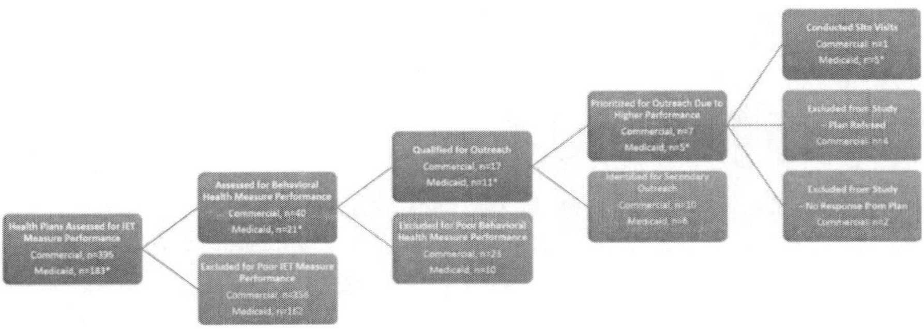

* One Medicaid health plan that did not appear in the NCQA data was included in the site visits due to their history of high performance and unique organizational and incentive structure.

Figure 8. Health Plan Site Visit Selection Process.

There was one exception to the aforementioned site selection process. The researchers chose to include a Northwest Medicaid plan that was not included in the NQCA data but had a history of high IET performance. Additionally, the researchers were familiar with this plan's organizational and incentive structure, which varied substantially from other Medicaid plans.

We included the plan in an initial list of 12 plans (seven commercial, five Medicaid) prioritized for outreach. See Figure 8 for a visual depiction of the site selection process.

Plan Recruitment

Initial outreach to health plans was via email. A standard, brief description of the study was included in each initial email message. We sent multiple follow-up emails to initially unresponsive plans. When contact was established, we made a follow-up phone call to explain the study and site visit request. In several cases, the initial health plan representative with whom we spoke requested to hold multiple follow-up calls with us and other health plan staff members to gain site visit approval. Many health plans never responded to our outreach emails, and some with whom we spoke ultimately declined to participate in the study (Figure 8). When a health plan did agree to participate in a site visit, we sent site visit agendas to the health plan contact describing which health plan representatives should be included in each group interview, and we used subsequent phone calls to clarify scheduling and participation. The researchers aimed to conduct six health plan site visits that included a mixture of commercial and Medicaid health plans.

We planned site visits to include multiple natural group interviews including health plan executives (e.g., Chief Executive Officer, Chief Operating Officer, Chief Marketing Officer), managers (e.g., Director of Quality, Director of Behavioral Health, Director of Contracting, Director of Care Management), and front-line providers (e.g., care managers). The researchers aimed to conduct separate group interviews for health plan executives and leadership, behavioral health teams, quality improvement teams, and care management teams in an effort to reproduce the natural social and team dynamics in which health plan staff operate.

Researchers anticipated that interviewee groupings would be based on the organizational structures of individual health plans. The researchers planned to design interview groupings in ways that would allow for: (1) duplicative questioning across different staffing groups; and (2) groups with common characteristics, such as health plan responsibilities or frequency of contact with plan beneficiaries, which would allow us to hone in on specific areas of interest.

Preliminary Data Collection

Preliminary Research

Researchers conducted preliminary research on health plans that were prioritized for site visits. Preliminary research included a limited Internet search of each health plan to identify basic plan information, including individuals in key leadership roles who should be included in outreach efforts. Once plans agreed to participate in preliminary calls to discuss the potential of study participation, the research team engaged in additional preliminary data collection.

Preliminary Calls

Preliminary calls with health plans expressing interest in participating in a site visit provided valuable insight on health plan organization and an overview of quality improvement initiatives. The researchers inquired about the governance structure of the health plans to better identify key informants for the site visit interviews. Additionally, the researchers asked health plan contacts to provide a brief, general overview of health plan quality improvement efforts that occurred during the performance period or were ongoing at the time of the call. We used this information to inform the interview group schedule and to frame researcher's semi-structured questions during the interviews.

Plan-Specific Environmental Scans

Prior to conducting the site visit, the research team performed a brief environmental scan of each health plan. These brief scans included reviews of the health plan website, plan publications including annual reports, and patient advisory reports. Such reviews yielded insight on health plan organizational structure, beneficiary population, and marketplace characteristics, including changes in Medicaid policy over time. The researchers also reviewed any recent news publications relevant to each plan.

Data Collection during Site Visits

Two research team members jointly conducted qualitative, semi-structured group interviews in person with health plan affiliates. Each interview lasted approximately 90 minutes, and there were multiple 90-minute interviews for each plan. Each interview included a group of health plan personnel or related stakeholders, with interview groupings determined on the basis of area of expertise and inquiry. One of the research team members recorded detailed descriptive notes during the interview, while the other team member conducted the interview using the prepared interview protocol and guide. Both the notetaker and the interviewer reviewed notes from each interview for accuracy. The data presented are from notes and may not reflect verbatim quotes from the interviewees.

Analytic Methods

We imported all interview notes into NVivo 11 (QSR International), a qualitative data management program. The qualitative project lead analyzed interviews using a thematic framework analysis approach in combination with more inductive strategies of grounded theory to enable novel themes to emerge within the analysis. To develop initial parent-code and subcode categories, we used constructs included in the theoretical model to explain participation in SUD treatment (Figure 1). The model describes four categories of factors hypothesized to affect initiation and engagement: (1) health plan factors; (2) market/environmental factors;

(3) individual patient-level factors; and (4) provider-level factors. Each of these four model components represented an original parent-code, populated with related subcodes. Using a partial grounded theory approach enabled the researchers to analyze the data inductively and to generate new theories about additional facilitators and barriers to initiation and engagement in SUD treatment that were not previously hypothesized in the conceptual framework. Through analysis, we identified multiple subcodes within the primary framework. We added one emergent parent-code to categorize comments specific to issues concerning IET measurement, including HEDIS criteria and costs associated with tracking and reporting on the HEDIS measures.

Consensus of the research team formed the basis for development of the initial codebook. One researcher used the codebook to systematically code interview notes. A senior researcher reviewed the coding. All coding discrepancies were reviewed by the research team and resolved by consensus decision. The inclusion of new codes and subcodes that emerged through the grounded approach also was conferred on and resolved by consensus within the research team. Appendix E provides the coding scheme that was developed.

RESULTS

Results of the quantitative and qualitative analyses are presented below. Because this is a mixed methods study in which quantitative results informed the subsequent qualitative analyses, the cross-cutting themes that emerged are elucidated in the Discussion section of this chapter.

Quantitative Results

We address below the results of analyses related to IET measures for SUD treatment and OUD treatment. Tables referenced below are at the end of the text describing the quantitative results for SUD treatment.

IET Measures for SUD Treatment

Plan Characteristics

A total of 321 health plans were included in the portion of the study that examined initiation and engagement in SUD treatment, with a mean beneficiary count of 50,585 (Table 10). The majority (62.3 percent) of the plans were PPOs. Thirty percent of the plans covered residential services for SUD. On average, the number of IOP outpatient or partial hospitalization SUD services provided per beneficiary was 0.005, and the mean number of SUD outpatient services was 0.008. Mean median provider reimbursement for outpatient SUD services was $186.25 per user and for inpatient SUD services was $6529.62 per user. Mean median out-of-pocket costs per user for outpatient services was $54.01, and costs per user for inpatient services was $980.20.

Plan Beneficiary Characteristics

On average, less than 0.5 percent of beneficiaries in these employer health plans had an identified SUD (Table 10). Approximately 55 percent of beneficiaries were between the ages of 18 and 44 years, and nearly 52 percent were female. Among those with an identified SUD, most (53.85 percent) did not use the emergency department, while 22.36 percent used it once, and 23.79 percent used it two times or more during the study period.

State-Level Market and Environmental Characteristics

Mean total state spending on the single state agency (SSA) for substance abuse services and state mental health per 1,000 members of the state population was $16,538.80 (Table 10). On average, the 67 percent of individuals in the states served by the plans identified as non-Hispanic White. Just under 20 percent lived below the poverty line and, on average, 66 percent of individuals in the states had private insurance. The mean past-year state prevalence rate of SUDs was slightly greater than 8 percent, with 7 percent aged 18 years and older receiving SUD treatment per 1,000 individuals in the state population.

Table 10. Characteristics of employer health plans included in the analysis of NCQA IET measures for SUD treatment (N=321)

Health Plan Characteristics	N	%	Mean
Number of beneficiaries	–	–	50584.60
Plan type			
PPO	200.00	62.30	–
HMO or capitated	60.00	18.70	–
High deductible	61.00	19.00	–
Reimbursement			
OP-OOP[a]	–	–	54.01
IP-OOP[b]	–	–	980.20
OP reimbursement[a]	–	–	186.25
IP reimbursement[b]	–	–	6529.62
Benefit design			
Residential	95.00	29.60	–
IOP/PH services	–	–	0.0047
OP services	–	–	0.0075
Beneficiary characteristics			
SUD beneficiaries	–	–	0.43
Age 18-44 years	–	–	55.06
Female	–	–	51.81
ED use			
0 times	–	–	53.85
1 time	–	–	22.36
2 or more times	–	–	23.79
Market characteristics			
SUD prevalence	–	–	8.38
SUD capacity	–	–	7.34
6 MAT medications	–	–	40.30
Non-Hispanic White	–	–	66.79
Poverty	–	–	19.87
Private insurance	–	–	66.01
PDMP	–	–	63.90
SSA spending	–	–	16358.80

Source: Truven Health MarketScan CCAE data, 2013-2014.

[a] Outpatient services include IOP services and partial hospitalization services in addition to other outpatient services.

[b] Inpatient services include inpatient and residential services.

Initiation variable skewness = -0.0627346; Initiation variable kurtosis = 0.27721992.

Engagement variable skewness = 0.85848228; Engagement variable kurtosis = 0.67542441.

Just over 40 percent of beneficiaries lived in states where all MAT medications for alcohol and OUDs were covered by Medicaid. Sixty-four percent lived in states that require prescribers or dispensers to access the state PDMP in certain circumstances.

Mean NCQA IET Measures by Health Plan Characteristics

The mean SUD treatment initiation rate for the health plans studied was 0.53, and the mean engagement rate was 0.14 (Table 11). Initiation and engagement rates did not differ greatly between plan types, although they tended to be somewhat lower in HMO or capitated plans than in either PPOs or high-deductible plans. Plans covering residential services had a marginally higher rate of initiation but not engagement. Plans that were equal to or above the mean in terms of numbers of IOP or partial hospitalization SUD services (initiation 0.58 vs 0.50; engagement 0.21 vs. 0.11) and SUD outpatient services (initiation 0.57 vs. 0.51; engagement 0.18 vs. 0.12) had higher initiation and engagement rates than plans that were below the mean in the provision of those services.

Similarly, those with higher median out-of-pocket costs for SUD outpatient services (initiation 0.55 vs. 0.51; engagement 0.15 vs. 0.14) and higher median provider reimbursement for outpatient SUD services (initiation 0.57 vs. 0.51; engagement 0.18 vs. 0.12) had higher initiation and engagement rates compared with those below the mean in out-of-pocket costs and provider reimbursement for outpatient SUD services. These findings on out-of-pocket cost (initiation 0.52 vs. 0.53; engagement 0.14 vs. 0.15) and reimbursement (initiation 0.52 vs. 0.53; engagement 0.14 vs. 0.15) were reversed for inpatient services.

Mean NCQA IET Measures by Plan Beneficiary Characteristics

In health plans with a mean or above mean percentage of beneficiaries with an identified SUD, the mean SUD treatment initiation rate (0.56 vs. 0.51) was higher, as was the mean engagement rate (0.16 vs. 0.13), compared with plans that had fewer of these beneficiaries (Table 11).

Table 11. Mean NCQA IET measures for SUD treatment by employer health plan characteristics (N=321)

Health Plan Characteristics	Initiation Rate Mean Rate	Engagement Rate Mean Rate
Measure rate	0.53	0.14
Plan type		
PPO	0.53	0.14
HMO or capitated	0.51	0.14
High deductible	0.52	0.14
Reimbursement		
OP-OOP[a]		
Plans equal to or above mean	0.55	0.15
Plans below mean	0.51	0.14
IP-OOP[b]		
Plans equal to or above mean	0.52	0.14
Plans below mean	0.53	0.15
OP reimbursement[a]		
Plans equal to or above mean	0.57	0.18
Plans below mean	0.51	0.12
IP reimbursement[b]		
Plans equal to or above mean	0.52	0.14
Plans below mean	0.53	0.15
Benefit design		
Residential	0.54	0.14
IOP/PH services		
Plans equal to or above mean	0.58	0.21
Plans below mean	0.50	0.11
OP services		
Plans equal to or above mean	0.57	0.18
Plans below mean	0.51	0.12
Beneficiary characteristics		
SUD beneficiaries		
Plans equal to or above mean	0.56	0.16
Plans below mean	0.51	0.13
Age 18-44 years		
Plans equal to or above mean	0.53	0.15
Plans below mean	0.53	0.13
Female		
Plans equal to or above mean	0.51	0.12

Table 11. (Continued)

Health Plan Characteristics	Initiation Rate Mean Rate	Engagement Rate Mean Rate
Plans below mean	0.54	0.16
ED use >2 times		
Plans equal to or above mean	0.53	0.14
Plans below mean	0.52	0.14
Market characteristics		
SUD prevalence		
Plans equal to or above mean	0.51	0.14
Plans below mean	0.55	0.14
SUD capacity		
Plans equal to or above mean	0.52	0.14
Plans below mean	0.53	0.14
Six MAT medications		
Plans equal to or above mean	0.54	0.14
Plans below mean	0.52	0.14
Non-Hispanic White		
Plans equal to or above mean	0.54	0.16
Plans below mean	0.51	0.13
Poverty		
Plans equal to or above mean	0.53	0.14
Plans below mean	0.53	0.15
Private insurance		
Plans equal to or above mean	0.55	0.16
Plans below mean	0.50	0.13
PDMP		
Plans equal to or above mean	0.53	0.15
Plans below mean	0.53	0.13
SSA spending		
Plans equal to or above mean	0.52	0.14
Plans below mean	0.53	0.15

Source: Truven Health MarketScan CCAE data, 2013-2014.

[a] Outpatient services include IOP services and partial hospitalization services in addition to other outpatient services.

[b] Inpatient services include inpatient and residential services.

There were few or no differences in rates related to emergency department use or age, although engagement rates were higher in plans where the percentage of beneficiaries aged 18-44 years was equal to or above the mean (0.15 vs. 0.13). Where the percentage of female beneficiaries was equal to or above the mean, rates of both initiation and engagement were lower (initiation 0.51 vs. 0.54; engagement 0.12 vs. 0.16).

Mean NCQA IET Measures by State-Level Market and Environmental Characteristics

Differences in initiation and engagement rates between plans equal to or above versus below the mean were minimal related to total state spending on the SSA, percentage of the population below the poverty line, and number of beneficiaries 18 years or older receiving SUD treatment relative to the state population (Table 11). However, when the state past-year prevalence of SUDs was equal to or above the mean, initiation rates were lower (0.51 vs. 0.55). In contrast, initiation rates were higher if a plan was in a state where all MAT medications for alcohol and OUDs were covered by Medicaid (0.54 vs. 0.52), a mean or above mean percentage of the population was non-Hispanic White (0.54 vs. 0.51), or a mean or above mean percentage of the population had private insurance (0.55 vs. 0.50). Engagement rates were higher if a plan was in a state where a mean or above mean percentage of the population was non-Hispanic White (0.16 vs. 0.13), a mean or above mean percentage of the population had private insurance (0.16 vs. 0.13), or where prescribers or dispensers were required to access the PDMP in certain circumstances (0.15 vs. 0.13).

Characteristics by Performance on the NCQA Initiation Measure

Health plans were divided into tertiles on the basis of performance on the initiation measure, with mean rates for the lowest tertile at 0.41, for the middle tertile 0.53, and for the highest tertile 0.64 (Table 12).

Compared with low performers, middle and high performers tended to be PPOs. Low performers were less apt to cover residential services and provided far fewer SUD IOP, partial hospitalization, or outpatient SUD services than did middle and high performers. The mean number of IOP or partial hospitalization services per beneficiary ranged from 0.0026 for low performers to 0.0075 for high performers, with the mean number of outpatient services ranging from 0.0051 for low performers to 0.0114 for high performers. Similarly, out-of-pocket outpatient costs were higher for high performers ($58.82) compared with low performers ($45.64), as was outpatient reimbursement ($244.87 vs. $161.79). Both inpatient out-of-pocket costs ($856.24 vs. $1055.87) and reimbursement to providers ($6248.28 vs. $7167.33) were far lower for plans that performed in the upper tertile compared with those in the lowest tertile.

Table 12. Employer health plan characteristics by performance on the NCQA initiation measure for SUD treatment (N=107)

Health Plan Characteristic	Lowest Tertile Performers N/Mean	Lowest Tertile Performers %	Middle Tertile Performers N/Mean	Middle Tertile Performers %	Highest Tertile Performers N/Mean	Highest Tertile Performers %
Initiation measure rate	0.41	–	0.53	–	0.64	–
Number of beneficiaries	46811.60	–	65667.40	–	39274.70	–
Plan type						
PPO	59.00	55.10	74.00	69.20	67.00	62.60
HMO or capitated	26.00	24.30	12.00	11.20	22.00	20.60
High deductible	22.00	20.60	21.00	19.60	18.00	16.80
Reimbursement						
OP-OOP[a]	45.64	–	57.56	–	58.82	–
IP-OOP[b]	1055.87	–	1028.50	–	856.24	–
OP reimbursement[a]	161.79	–	152.10	–	244.87	–
IP reimbursement[b]	7167.33	–	6173.26	–	6248.28	–
Benefit design						
Residential	27.00	25.20	37.00	34.60	31.00	29.00
IOP/PH services	0.0026	–	0.0039	–	0.0075	–
OP services	0.0051	–	0.0061	–	0.0114	–
Beneficiary characteristics						
SUD beneficiaries	0.39	–	0.38	–	0.52	–
Age 18-44 years	55.25	–	56.61	–	53.33	–
Female	52.02	–	51.81	–	51.59	–
ED use						
0 times	54.91	–	53.33	–	53.32	–
1 time	21.85	–	22.86	–	22.36	–
2 or more times	23.25	–	23.81	–	24.32	–
Market characteristics						
SUD prevalence	8.42	–	8.37	–	8.34	–
SUD capacity	7.46	–	7.46	–	7.10	–
6 MAT medications	43.15	–	33.92	–	43.83	–
Non-Hispanic White	62.90	–	66.89	–	70.57	–

Health Plan Characteristic	Lowest Tertile Performers N/Mean	Lowest Tertile Performers %	Middle Tertile Performers N/Mean	Middle Tertile Performers %	Highest Tertile Performers N/Mean	Highest Tertile Performers %
Poverty	19.71	–	20.06	–	19.83	–
Private insurance	65.22	–	65.58	–	67.24	–
PDMP	61.39	–	67.94	–	62.36	–
SSA spending	17307.40	–	15781.50	–	15987.50	–

Source: Truven Health MarketScan CCAE data, 2013-2014.

[a] Outpatient services include IOP services and partial hospitalization services in addition to other outpatient services.

[b] Inpatient services include inpatient and residential services.

Compared with the lowest performing plans, plans that were highest performing on initiation had more beneficiaries identified with SUDs (0.52 percent vs. 0.39 percent) (Table 12). They also had lower percentages of beneficiaries aged 18-44 years (53.33 percent vs. 55.25 percent). The most pronounced market or environmental characteristics that differed between the lowest and highest tertile plans were: (1) mean total state spending on the SSA (higher for low performing plans); (2) mean percentage of individuals in the state who were non-Hispanic White (lower for low performing plans); and (3) mean percentage of individuals in the state with private insurance (lower for low performing plans).

Characteristics by Performance on the NCQA Engagement Measure

Health plans also were divided into tertiles on the engagement measure for SUD services, with mean rates for the lowest tertile at 0.05, the middle tertile at 0.13, and the highest tertile at 0.25 (Table 13). The lowest performing plans had the highest mean number of beneficiaries. Middle and high tertile plans were PPOs to a greater extent than were low performing plans. There were no substantial differences in initiation rates depending on the provision of residential SUD services by the plans. The mean number of IOP or partial hospitalization services per beneficiary ranged from 0.0021 for low performers to 0.0083 for high performers, with the mean number of outpatient services ranging from 0.0051 for low performers to 0.0117 for high performers.

Table 13. Employer health plan characteristics by performance on the NCQA engagement measure for SUD treatment (N=107)

Health Plan Characteristic	Lowest Tertile Performers N/Mean	Lowest Tertile Performers %	Middle Tertile Performers N/Mean	Middle Tertile Performers %	Highest Tertile Performers N/Mean	Highest Tertile Performers %
Engagement measure rate	0.05	–	0.13	–	0.25	–
Number of beneficiaries	56568.50	–	49913.70	–	45271.50	–
Plan type						
PPO	57.00	53.30	77.00	72.00	66.00	61.70
HMO or capitated	29.00	27.10	11.00	10.30	20.00	18.70
High deductible	21.00	19.60	19.00	17.80	21.00	19.60
Reimbursement						
OP-OOP[a]	50.72	–	55.57	–	55.73	–
IP-OOP[b]	996.45	–	979.12	–	965.03	–
OP reimbursement[a]	137.50	–	150.06	–	271.19	–
IP reimbursement[b]	7239.56	–	6081.28	–	6268.03	–
Benefit design						
Residential	31.00	29.00	32.00	29.90	32.00	29.90
IOP/PH services	0.0021	–	0.0034	–	0.0083	–
OP services	0.0051	–	0.0058	–	0.0117	–
Beneficiary characteristics						
SUD beneficiaries	0.41	–	0.41	–	0.47	–
Age 18-44 years	54.98	–	54.38	–	55.83	–
Female	52.11	–	52.70	–	50.61	–
ED use						
0 times	53.84	–	53.77	–	53.94	–
1 time	22.45	–	22.66	–	21.96	–
2 or more times	23.71	–	23.57	–	24.10	–
Market characteristics						
SUD prevalence	8.42	–	8.30	–	8.41	–
SUD capacity	8.01	–	6.83	–	7.19	–
6 MAT medications	45.83	–	34.99	–	40.07	–

Health Plan Characteristic	Lowest Tertile Performers N/Mean	Lowest Tertile Performers %	Middle Tertile Performers N/Mean	Middle Tertile Performers %	Highest Tertile Performers N/Mean	Highest Tertile Performers %
Non-Hispanic White	62.76	–	67.67	–	69.94	–
Poverty	19.88	–	20.08	–	19.64	–
Private insurance	65.16	–	65.96	–	66.92	–
PDMP	60.94	–	64.39	–	66.36	–
SSA spending	17040.60	–	15534.40	–	16501.50	–

Source: Truven Health MarketScan CCAE data, 2013-2014.

[a] Outpatient services include IOP services and partial hospitalization services in addition to other outpatient services.

[b] Inpatient services include inpatient and residential services.

Differences in reimbursement characteristics were greatest for median provider reimbursement for outpatient SUD services per user (low performing $137.50 vs. high $271.19), for median provider reimbursement for inpatient SUD services per user (low performing $7239.56 vs. high $6268.03), and for median out-of-pocket costs for inpatient SUD services per user (low performing $996.45 vs. high $965.03).

Major differences in beneficiary characteristics were not seen between plans at different levels of performance (Table 13). Compared with middle performing plans, market and environmental characteristics often were more similar between low and high performing plans. However, the highest tertile performers also had higher percentages of beneficiaries living in states requiring prescribers or dispensers to access the PDMP (low performing 60.94 percent vs. high 66.36 percent) and higher percentages of individuals living in states with a higher percentage of non-Hispanic White population (high performing 69.94 percent vs. 62.76 percent).

Table 14. Multivariate regression results examining the effect of health plan and environmental characteristics on employer health plan performance on the NCQA IET measures for SUD treatment (N=321)

Health Plan Characteristics	Initiation Measure Beta	Initiation Measure p-value	Engagement Measure Beta	Engagement Measure p-value
Number of beneficiaries	6.21E-08	0.4523	-4.1E-09	0.9528
Plan type				
PPO	Reference	Reference	Reference	Reference
HMO or capitated	-0.01858	0.2345	-0.00948	0.4723
High deductible	-0.00244	0.8674	-0.00386	0.7541
Reimbursement				
OP-OOP[a]	0.000517	0.0007	9.13E-05	0.4774
IP-OOP[b]	-9.8E-06	0.1948	-4.5E-06	0.4846
OP reimbursement[a]	-1.1E-05	0.6301	2.8E-06	0.8869
IP reimbursement[b]	1.92E-06	0.2331	3.42E-07	0.8014
Benefit design				
Residential	0.0101	0.409	0.000302	0.9766
IOP/PH services	2.06408	0.0103	3.82326	<0.0001
OP services	1.45792	0.1467	4.13869	<0.0001
Beneficiary characteristics				
SUD beneficiaries	7.43985	0.0573	-12.6598	0.0001
Age 18-44 years	-0.01623	0.7253	-0.00937	0.8102
Female	-0.07323	0.5486	-0.20293	0.0497
ED use				
0 times	Reference	Reference	Reference	Reference
1 time	0.14589	0.2275	-0.12134	0.2347
2 or more times	-0.11496	0.192	-0.08526	0.2518
Market characteristics				
SUD prevalence	-0.00705	0.68	0.00706	0.6247
SUD capacity	-0.00071	0.5954	-0.00138	0.2233
Six MAT medications	0.00639	0.763	-0.00641	0.7201
Non-Hispanic White	0.00248	0.0001	0.0017	0.0019
Poverty	0.00178	0.5746	0.000502	0.8514
PDMP	-0.02494	0.2341	0.01716	0.3322
SSA spending	-1.5E-06	0.172	1.56E-07	0.8691

Source: Truven Health MarketScan CCAE data, 2013-2014.

[a] Outpatient services include IOP services and partial hospitalization services in addition to other outpatient services.

[b] Inpatient services include inpatient and residential services. Initiation measure regression r^2: 0.2609. Engagement measure regression r^2: 0.3476.

Results of Multivariate analysis on Characteristics Influencing Initiation and Engagement

Characteristics significantly associated with higher rates of SUD treatment initiation among employer health plans included providing higher numbers of IOP and partial hospitalization services per beneficiary ($\beta = 2.06408$, $p = 0.0103$), having higher than the mean median out-of-pocket costs for outpatient SUD services per user ($\beta = 0.000517$, $p = 0.0007$), and being in a state with a higher percentage of individuals who were non-Hispanic White ($\beta = 0.00248$, $p = 0.0001$). (Table 14).

Higher rates of SUD treatment engagement were associated with: (1) providing higher numbers of SUD IOP and partial hospitalization services per beneficiary ($\beta = 3.82326$, $p < 0.0001$); (2) providing higher numbers of SUD outpatient services per beneficiary ($\beta = 4.13869$, $p < 0.0001$); and (3) being in a state with a higher percentage of individuals who were non-Hispanic White ($\beta = 0.0017$, $p = 0.0019$). Higher rates of engagement were negatively associated with having more beneficiaries in the plan with an identified SUD ($\beta = -12.6598$, $p = 0.0001$) and more beneficiaries who are female ($\beta = -0.20293$, $p = 0.0497$).

IET Measures for OUD Treatment

Plan Characteristics

A total of 82 health plans were included in the portion of the study that examined initiation and engagement rates for those with identified OUDs, with a mean beneficiary count of 92,521 (Table 15). The majority (66 percent) of the plans were PPOs.

Approximately 37 percent of the plans covered residential services. On average, the number of IOP or partial hospitalization SUD services provided per beneficiary was 0.005 and the mean number of SUD outpatient services was 0.009. Among those beneficiaries with identified OUD, 53 percent did not receive MAT, 3 percent received it for 14 days or less, and 44 percent received it for more than 14 days. Mean median provider reimbursement for outpatient SUD services was $181.83 per user, for inpatient SUD services was $5656.22 per user, and for MAT was

$2292.98 per user. Mean median out-of-pocket cost per user for outpatient services was $47.51, mean median cost per user for inpatient services was $767.80, and mean median cost per user for MAT medications was $302.26.

Plan Beneficiary Characteristics

On average, less than 0.29 percent of beneficiaries in these employer health plans had an identified OUD (Table 15). Approximately 54 percent of beneficiaries were between the ages of 18 and 44 years, and nearly 52 percent were female. Among those with an SUD, most (55.6 percent) did not use the emergency department, while 20.7 percent used it once, and 23.7 percent used it two times or more during the study period.

State-Level Market and Environmental Characteristics

For this smaller subset of health plans, mean total state spending on the SSA per 1,000 members of the state population was $16,325.90 (Table 15). On average, 68 percent of individuals in the states served by the plans identified as being non-Hispanic White. Just over 20 percent lived below the poverty line and, on average, 66 percent of individuals in the state had private insurance. The mean past-year state prevalence rate of opioid prescriptions was 93.5 per 100 individuals in the state, with 7 percent aged 18 years and older receiving SUD treatment per 1,000 individuals in the state population. Fifty-two percent of beneficiaries lived in states where all three MAT medications for OUD were covered by Medicaid. Sixty-eight percent lived in states that require prescribers or dispensers to access the state PDMP in certain circumstances. There were approximately 144 OTP spaces available for methadone per 100,000 population in the states, and the mean number of buprenorphine prescribers per 100,000 population was eight.

Table 15. Characteristics of employer health plans included in the analysis of NCQA IET measures, limited to OUDs (N=82)

Health Plan Characteristic	N	%	Mean
Number of beneficiaries	–	–	92521.10
Plan type			
PPO	54.00	65.90	–
HMO or capitated	16.00	19.50	–
High deductible	12.00	14.60	–
Reimbursement			
MAT OOP	–	–	302.26
OP-OOP[a]	–	–	47.51
IP-OOP[b]	–	–	767.80
MAT reimbursement	–	–	2292.98
OP reimbursement[a]	–	–	181.83
IP reimbursement[b]	–	–	5656.22
Benefit design			
MAT use			
None	–	–	0.53
14 days or less	–	–	0.03
>14 days	–	–	0.44
Residential	30.00	36.60	–
IOP/PH services	–	–	0.0053
OP services	–	–	0.0090
Beneficiary characteristics			
OUD beneficiaries	–	–	0.29
Age 18-44 years	–	–	53.90
Female	–	–	51.91
ED use			
0 times	–	–	55.61
1 time	–	–	20.65
2 or more times	–	–	23.74
Market characteristics			
Opioid prescriptions	–	–	93.46
SUD capacity	–	–	7.21
OTP capacity	–	–	143.63
Buprenorphine prescribers	–	–	8.26
3 MAT	–	–	52.00
Non-Hispanic White	–	–	68.27
Poverty	–	–	20.33
Private insurance	–	–	66.11
PDMP	–	–	67.95
SSA spending	–	–	16325.90

Source: Truven Health MarketScan CCAE data, 2013-2014.

[a] Outpatient services include IOP services and partial hospitalization services in addition to other outpatient services.

[b] Inpatient services include inpatient and residential services.

Initiation variable skewness = 0.47826139; Initiation variable kurtosis = 0.16101831.

Engagement variable skewness = 0.51762313; Engagement variable kurtosis = -0.2974445.

Mean NCQA IET Measures by Health Plan Characteristics

The mean initiation rate for OUD treatment for the health plans was 0.55, and the mean engagement rate for OUD treatment was 0.15 (Table 16). Both initiation and engagement rates tended to be higher in PPO plans, particularly compared with high deductible plans (initiation 0.56 vs. 0.51; engagement 0.16 vs. 0.13). Plans covering residential services had a slightly higher rate of initiation (0.57) and engagement (0.16) compared with the mean per plan. Plans that were equal to or above the mean in terms of numbers of IOP or partial hospitalization SUD services (initiation 0.61 vs 0.51; engagement (0.20 vs. 0.13) and SUD outpatient services (initiation 0.60 vs. 0.52; engagement vs. 0.13) had higher initiation and engagement rates than plans that were below the mean in the provision of those services. Plans that were above the mean percentage of beneficiaries with OUDs who received MAT in excess of 14 days did not have higher initiation rates compared with plans with a lower percentage of beneficiaries meeting these characteristics who did have higher engagement rates (0.17 vs. 0.13). Compared with plans below the mean in out-of-pocket costs and provider reimbursement for outpatient services, plans with higher median out-of-pocket costs for SUD outpatient services had marginally lower initiation rates but higher engagement rates (initiation 0.54 vs. 0.55; engagement 0.16 vs. 0.15), and plans with higher median provider reimbursement for outpatient SUD services (initiation 0.58 vs. 0.53; engagement 0.19 vs. 0.13) had higher initiation and engagement rates. Health plans with mean or above mean out-of-pocket costs (initiation 0.53 vs. 0.56; engagement 0.14 vs. 0.17) or provider reimbursement (initiation 0.54 vs. 0.55; engagement 0.14 vs. 0.16) for inpatient services had lower rates for both initiation and engagement. Health plans that had mean or above mean pharmacy reimbursement for MAT showed both higher initiation (0.58 vs. 0.52) and engagement (0.16 vs. 0.15) rates compared with those with pharmacy reimbursement below the mean. When median out-of-pocket costs were equal to or above the mean for MAT medications, initiation rates were lower (0.53 vs. 0.56) and engagement rates higher (0.16 vs. 0.15) compared with plans with lower out-of-pocket costs.

Table 16. Mean NCQA IET measures by employer health plan characteristics, limited to OUDs (N=41)

Health Plan Characteristic	Initiation Rate Mean Rate	Engagement Rate Mean Rate
Measure rate	0.55	0.15
Plan type		
PPO	0.56	0.16
HMO or capitated	0.53	0.15
High deductible	0.51	0.13
Reimbursement		
MAT OOP		
Plans equal to or above mean	0.53	0.16
Plans below mean	0.56	0.15
OP-OOP[a]		
Plans equal to or above mean	0.54	0.16
Plans below mean	0.55	0.15
IP-OOP[b]		
Plans equal to or above mean	0.53	0.14
Plans below mean	0.56	0.17
MAT reimbursement		
Plans equal to or above mean	0.58	0.16
Plans below mean	0.52	0.15
OP reimbursement[a]		
Plans equal to or above mean	0.58	0.19
Plans below mean	0.53	0.13
Median provider reimbursement for inpatient SUD services[b]		
Plans equal to or above mean	0.54	0.14
Plans below mean	0.55	0.16
Benefit design		
MAT use >14 days		
Plans equal to or above mean	0.55	0.17
Plans below mean	0.55	0.13
Residential services	0.57	0.16
IOP/PH services		
Plans equal to or above mean	0.61	0.20
Plans below mean	0.51	0.13
OP services		
Plans equal to or above mean	0.60	0.20
Plans below mean	0.52	0.13

Table 16. (Continued)

Health Plan Characteristic	**Initiation Rate Mean Rate**	**Engagement Rate Mean Rate**
Beneficiary characteristics		
OUD beneficiaries		
Plans equal to or above mean	0.58	0.15
Plans below mean	0.52	0.15
Age 18-44 years		
Plans equal to or above mean	0.54	0.17
Plans below mean	0.55	0.14
Female		
Plans equal to or above mean	0.52	0.12
Plans below mean	0.57	0.18
ED use 2 times or more		
Plans equal to or above mean	0.58	0.17
Plans below mean	0.52	0.13
Market characteristics		
Opioid prescriptions		
Plans equal to or above mean	0.59	0.18
Plans below mean	0.51	0.13
SUD capacity		
Plans equal to or above mean	0.51	0.14
Plans below mean	0.57	0.16
OTP capacity		
Plans equal to or above mean	0.53	0.14
Plans below mean	0.56	0.16
Buprenorphine prescribers		
Plans equal to or above mean	0.55	0.16
Plans below mean	0.54	0.15
3 MAT medications		
Plans equal to or above mean	0.59	0.17
Plans below mean	0.52	0.14
Non-Hispanic White		
Plans equal to or above mean	0.59	0.18
Plans below mean	0.52	0.13
Poverty		
Plans equal to or above mean	0.55	0.15
Plans below mean	0.54	0.16

Health Plan Characteristic	Initiation Rate Mean Rate	Engagement Rate Mean Rate
Private insurance		
Plans equal to or above mean	0.59	0.17
Plans below mean	0.50	0.13
PDMP		
Plans equal to or above mean	0.52	0.15
Plans below mean	0.58	0.16
SSA spending		
Plans equal to or above mean	0.55	0.16
Plans below mean	0.54	0.14

Source: Truven Health MarketScan CCAE data, 2013-2014.

[a] Outpatient services include IOP services and partial hospitalization services in addition to other outpatient services.

[b] Inpatient services include inpatient and residential services.

Mean NCQA IET Measures by Plan Beneficiary Characteristics

In health plans with a mean or above mean percentage of beneficiaries with an identified OUD, the mean initiation rate (0.58 vs. 0.52) was higher compared with plans with fewer beneficiaries with these characteristics, while there were no differences for engagement (Table 16). Both initiation (0.58 vs. 0.52) and engagement (0.17 vs. 0.13) rates were higher in plans with mean to above mean percentages of beneficiaries with OUD who used the emergency department two or more times. Engagement rates were higher in plans where the percentage of beneficiaries aged 18-44 years was equal to or above the mean (0.17 vs. 0.14). Where the percentage of female beneficiaries was equal to or above mean, rates of both initiation and engagement were lower (initiation 0.52 vs. 0.57; engagement 0.12 vs. 0.18).

Mean NCQA IET Measures by State-Level Market and Environmental Characteristics

Initiation and engagement rates for OUD treatment were somewhat higher for plans in states where total state spending on the SSA was equal to or above the mean (initiation 0.55 vs. 0.54; engagement 0.16 vs. 0.14) and where the number of buprenorphine prescribers per 100,000 state population was equal to or above the mean (initiation 0.55 vs. 0.54; engagement 0.16 vs. 0.15) (Table 16). Both rates were quite a bit higher for plans in states that were equal to or above the mean for prevalence of opioid prescriptions per 100 people (initiation 0.59 vs. 0.51; engagement 0.18 vs. 0.13), states where all three OUD MAT medications were covered by Medicaid (initiation 0.59 vs. 0.52; engagement 0.17 vs. 0.14), where the percentage of the non-Hispanic White population was higher (initiation 0.59 vs. 0.52; engagement 0.18 vs. 0.13), and where more of the population had private insurance (initiation 0.59 vs. 0.50; engagement 0.17 vs. 0.13). Where the number of beneficiaries aged 18 or older receiving SUD treatment per 1,000 population was at or above mean, both initiation and engagement rates were lower (initiation 0.51 vs. 0.57; engagement 0.14 vs. 0.16); the same was true where the number of OTP spaces for methadone was greater (initiation 0.53 vs. 0.56; engagement 0.14 vs. 0.16).

Similarly, both initiation and engagement rates were lower if a plan was in a state where prescribers or dispensers were required to access the PDMP in certain circumstances (initiation 0.52 vs. 0.58; engagement 0.15 vs. 0.16).

Characteristics by Performance on the NCQA Initiation Measure

Health plans were divided into low and high performers on the basis of rates of OUD initiation, with mean initiation rates for low performers of 0.50 and for high performers of 0.59 (Table 17). Low performers tended to have a greater number of beneficiaries (118,862 on average), compared with high performers (66,180 on average). High performers were more often PPOs (71 percent) than were low performers (61 percent). Low performers were less apt to cover residential services and provided far fewer SUD IOP, partial hospitalization, or outpatient SUD services than did high performers. The mean number of IOP or partial hospitalization services per beneficiary ranged from 0.0036 for low performers to 0.0071 for high performers, with the mean number of outpatient services ranging from 0.0067 for low performers to 0.0114 for high performers. Higher percentages of those with OUDs received MAT for longer than 14 days (47 percent) compared with low performers (42 percent). Out-of-pocket inpatient costs were lower for high performers ($914.44 vs. $621.15), as was provider reimbursement for inpatient SUD services ($5790.96 vs.

$5521.48). Out-of-pocket costs for MAT medications ($301.91 vs. $302.61) and pharmacy reimbursement for MAT medications ($2187.43 vs. 2398.52) also were lower for low performers compared with high performers on the initiation measure. Out-of-pocket outpatient costs were lower for high performers ($45.16) compared with low performers ($49.86), whereas outpatient reimbursement showed higher rates for high performers ($147.78 vs. $215.88).

Compared with the lowest performing plans, plans that were highest performing on initiation had more beneficiaries identified with OUDs (0.33 percent vs. 0.26 percent) (Table 17). They also had higher percentages of beneficiaries between the ages of 18 and 44 years (54.67 percent vs. 53.14 percent) and higher percentages of beneficiaries who used the emergency department two or more times (24.69 vs. 22.79). Higher-performing plans had fewer beneficiaries who were female (50.33 vs. 53.48). Market and environmental characteristics with little distinction between a low and high performing plan included level of poverty in the state, private insurance penetration in the state, and availability of buprenorphine providers in the state, although the latter was somewhat higher for high performing plans (8.55 vs. 7.98).

The high performers did have more beneficiaries in states with high prevalence of opioid prescriptions (99.58 vs. 87.33 per 100 population), coverage of all three OUD MAT medications (57.47 percent vs. 46.54 percent), and populations with higher percentages of non-Hispanic White individuals (71.60 percent vs. 64.95 percent). High performing plans had a lower mean number of beneficiaries aged 18 years or older receiving SUD treatment (6.19 vs. 8.23 per 1,000 population), lower numbers of OTP spaces available for methadone (127.54 vs. 159.72, per 100,000 population), less money spent on the state SSA per person ($15,300.00 vs. $17,351.80), and fewer beneficiaries living in states requiring prescribers or dispensers to access the PDMP (61.90 percent vs. 74.00 percent).

Table 17. Employer health plan characteristics by performance on the NCQA initiation measure, limited to OUDs (N=41)

Health Plan Characteristic	Low Performers N/Mean	Low Performers %	High Performers N/Mean	High Performers %
Initiation measure rate	0.50	–	0.59	–
Number of beneficiaries	118862.00	–	66180.00	–
Plan type				
PPO	25.00	61.00	29.00	70.70
HMO or capitated	9.00	22.00	7.00	17.10
High deductible	7.00	17.10	5.00	12.20
Reimbursement				
MAT OOP	301.91	–	302.61	–
OP-OOP[a]	49.86	–	45.16	–
IP-OOP[b]	914.44	–	621.15	–
MAT reimbursement	2187.43	–	2398.52	–
OP reimbursement[a]	147.78	–	215.88	–
IP reimbursement[b]	5790.96	–	5521.48	–
Benefit design				
MAT use				
None	56.00	–	50.00	–
14 days or less	2.00	–	3.00	–
>14 days	42.00	–	47.00	–
Residential	14.00	34.10	16.00	39.00
IOP/PH services	0.0036	–	0.0071	–
OP services	0.0067	–	0.0114	–
Beneficiary characteristics				
OUD beneficiaries	0.26	–	0.33	–
Age 18-44 years	53.14	–	54.67	–
Female	53.48	–	50.33	–
ED use				
0 times	57.10	–	54.12	–
1 time	20.10	–	21.19	–
2 or more times	22.79	–	24.69	–
Market characteristics				
Opioid prescriptions	87.33	–	99.58	–
SUD capacity	8.23	–	6.19	–
OTP capacity	159.72	–	127.54	–
Buprenorphine prescribers	7.98	–	8.55	–
3 MAT	46.54	–	57.47	–
Non-Hispanic White	64.95	–	71.60	–
Poverty	20.32	–	20.33	–
Private insurance	65.24	–	66.99	–
PDMP	74.00	–	61.90	–
SSA spending	17351.80	–	15300.00	–

Source: Truven Health MarketScan CCAE data, 2013-2014.

[a] Outpatient services include IOP services and partial hospitalization services in addition to other outpatient services.

[b] Inpatient services include inpatient and residential services.

Characteristics by Performance on the NCQA Engagement Measure

Health plans also were divided into high and low performers on OUD engagement, with mean rates of 0.10 for the low performers and 0.21 for the high performers (Table 18). The lowest performing plans for engagement also had the highest mean number of beneficiaries. Seventy-six percent of high performing plans were PPOs, compared with 56 percent of low performing plans. Residential SUD treatment was provided by a higher percentage of high performing plans (42 percent) compared with low performers (32 percent). The mean number of IOP or partial hospitalization services per beneficiary ranged from 0.0031 for low performers to 0.0075 for high performers, with the mean number of outpatient services ranging from 0.0061 for low performers to 0.0120 for high performers. Compared with low performing plans, high performers were more likely to have beneficiaries with OUD who received MAT for more than 14 days (low performing 41 percent vs. high 48 percent). Differences in reimbursement characteristics were largest for median provider reimbursement for inpatient SUD services per user (low performing $5758.57 vs. high $5553.86), median out-of-pocket costs for inpatient SUD services per user (low performing $890.25 vs. $645.35), and median provider reimbursement for outpatient SUD services per user (low performing $136.31 vs. high performing $227.34). Median outpatient SUD out-of-pocket costs also were higher for high performing plans, but out-of-pocket costs for MAT were lower for high performing plans, as was pharmacy reimbursement for MAT.

Major differences in beneficiary characteristics were not seen between plans at different levels of performance, although high performing plans had higher percentages of beneficiaries with an identified OUD, had more beneficiaries with OUD using the emergency department two or more times, more beneficiaries between the ages of 18-44 years, and fewer beneficiaries who were female.

Table 18. Employer health plan characteristics by performance on the NCQA engagement measure, limited for OUDs (N=41)

Health Plan Characteristic	Low Performers N/Mean	Low Performers %	High Performers N/Mean	High Performers %
Engagement measure	0.10	–	0.21	–
Number of beneficiaries	115244.00	–	69797.80	–
Plan type				
PPO	23.00	56.10	31.00	75.60
HMO or capitated	10.00	24.40	6.00	14.60
High deductible	8.00	19.50	4.00	9.80
Reimbursement				
MAT OOP	304.42	–	300.10	–
OP-OOP[a]	46.30	–	48.71	–
IP-OOP[b]	890.25	–	645.35	–
MAT reimbursement	2300.95	–	2285.01	–
OP reimbursement[a]	136.31	–	227.34	–
IP reimbursement[b]	5758.57	–	5553.86	–
Benefit design				
MAT use				
None	57.00	–	49.00	–
14 days or less	2.00	–	3.00	–
>14 days	41.00	–	48.00	–
Residential	13.00	31.70	17.00	41.50
IOP/PH services	0.0031	–	0.0075	–
OP services	0.0061	–	0.0120	–
Beneficiary characteristics				
OUD beneficiaries	0.27	–	0.31	–
Age 18-44 years	52.29	–	55.52	–
Female	53.28	–	50.53	–
ED use				
0 times	56.87	–	54.36	–
1 time	20.22	–	21.08	–
2 or more times	22.92	–	24.57	–
Market characteristics				
Opioid prescriptions	93.29	–	93.63	–
SUD capacity	7.88	–	6.54	–
OTP capacity	151.28	–	135.99	–
Buprenorphine prescribers	7.95	–	8.58	–
3 MAT	52.41	–	51.59	–
Non-Hispanic White	65.71	–	70.84	–
Poverty	20.75	–	19.90	–

Health Plan Characteristic	Low Performers N/Mean	Low Performers %	High Performers N/Mean	High Performers %
Private insurance	65.21	–	67.02	–
PDMP	69.36	–	66.54	–
SSA spending	16110.90	–	16540.90	–

Source: Truven Health MarketScan CCAE data, 2013-2014.

[a] Outpatient services include IOP services and partial hospitalization services in addition to other outpatient services.

[b] Inpatient services include inpatient and residential services.

Examination of market and environmental characteristics revealed that the factors most strongly differentiating low from high performing plans on the engagement measure for OUD treatment were that high performing plans were most often in states that spent more on the SSA per state population (low performing $16,110.90 vs. high $16,540.90), were less likely to be in states where prescribers or dispensers are required to access the PDMP (low performing 69.36 percent vs high 66.54 percent), had fewer OTP spaces for methadone (low performing 151.28 vs. high 135.99 per 100,000 population), had higher numbers of non-Hispanic White individuals in the population (low performing 65.71 percent vs. high 70.84 percent), and had higher numbers of individuals in the state with private insurance (low performing 65.21 percent vs. high 67.02 percent).

Results of Multivariate Analysis on Characteristics Influencing Initiation and Engagement

Characteristics significantly associated with higher rates of initiation of OUD treatment among employer health plans included providing higher numbers of IOP and partial hospitalization services per beneficiary (β = 4.47344, p = 0.0409) and being in a state with above mean prevalence of opioid prescriptions per 100 people in the state (β = 0.00228, p = 0.024) (Table 19). Negative associations also were seen, including higher rates of initiation of OUD treatment negatively associated with being in a state where prescribers or dispensers are required to access the PDMP under certain circumstances (β = -0.0864, p = 0.0362).

Table 19. Multivariate regression results examining the effect of health plan and environmental characteristics on employer health plan performance on the NCQA IET measures, limited to OUDs (N=82)

Health Plan Characteristics	Initiation Measure Beta	Initiation Measure p-value	Engagement Measure Beta	Engagement Measure p-value
Number of beneficiaries	2.16E-08	0.7804	-4.4E-08	0.2267
Plan type				
PPO	Reference	Reference	Reference	Reference
HMO or capitated	0.01573	0.4804	-0.00602	0.5628
High deductible	0.0022	0.922	-0.01354	0.2006
Reimbursement				
MAT OOP	-1.5E-06	0.98	1.16E-05	0.6735
OP-OOP[a]	0.000373	0.1497	0.000139	0.2494
IP-OOP[b]	-1.1E-05	0.4726	-5E-06	0.4841
MAT reimbursement	-7.7E-06	0.6506	1.53E-06	0.8475
OP reimbursement[a]	0.000129	0.1579	8.18E-05	0.057
IP reimbursement[b]	-7.8E-07	0.8422	1.01E-06	0.5826
Benefit design				
MAT use				
None	Reference	Reference	Reference	Reference
14 days or less	0.52499	0.1406	0.22302	0.179
>14 days	0.05631	0.5172	0.03338	0.4114
Residential	0.00705	0.6487	0.00124	0.8637
IOP/PH services	4.47344	0.0409	4.07017	0.0001
OP services	-1.0704	0.5242	-0.57529	0.4635
Beneficiary characteristics				
OUD beneficiaries	0.34887	0.9667	-10.549	0.0089
Age 18-44 years	-0.04029	0.5353	-0.02013	0.507
Female	-0.27617	0.13	-0.1958	0.0233
ED use				
0 times	Reference	Reference	Reference	Reference
1 time	0.12579	0.5519	0.01033	0.9165
2 or more times	-0.03954	0.7857	-0.0384	0.572
Market characteristics				
Opioid prescriptions	0.00228	0.024	-0.00013	0.7705
SUD capacity	0.00013	0.4067	-9.1E-05	0.2132
OTP capacity	0.00567	0.3107	0.00221	0.3977
Buprenorphine prescribers	-0.07678	0.0352	-0.03747	0.028
3 MAT	0.000122	0.948	0.000873	0.3197
Non-Hispanic White	-0.00541	0.4227	-0.0006	0.8484
PDMP	-0.0864	0.0362	0.00574	0.761
SSA spending	-8.2E-07	0.8013	1.35E-06	0.3756

Source: Truven Health MarketScan CCAE data, 2013-2014.

[a] Outpatient services include IOP services and partial hospitalization services in addition to other outpatient services.

[b] Inpatient services include inpatient and residential services. Initiation measure regression r^2: 0.6101.

Engagement measure regression r^2: 0.6625.

Higher rates of engagement were associated with providing higher numbers of SUD IOP and partial hospitalization services per beneficiary ($\beta = 4.07017$, $p = 0.0001$). Negative associations also were seen, such as higher rates of engagement negatively associated with having a higher percentage of beneficiaries with an identified OUD ($\beta = -10.549$, $p = 0.0089$) or having a higher percentage of beneficiaries who are female ($\beta = -0.1958$, $p = 0.0233$).

Qualitative Results

Plan Characteristics

Six health plans participated in site visit interviews – five Medicaid plans and one commercial plan. The plans served geographically diverse populations across the United States. Two plans served Western states, two plans covered Midwestern states, one served a Northeastern state, and one served a Southeastern state. Health plans described covering diverse populations, including urban and rural populations. They varied substantially in the size of their membership, ranging from approximately 9,880 to 2.9 million covered lives.

Group interviews with health plans included plan representatives in varying roles – from executive leadership to quality improvement strategy teams to clinicians and other staff members engaged in beneficiary outreach efforts. The research team interviewed a total of 65 health plan stakeholders, averaging 11 individuals per plan. To obtain information regarding health plan governance, organization, culture, and strategy from key systems leaders, across all site visits the researchers interviewed two health plan presidents; eight chief executive officers, operating officers, or other individuals in operations leadership positions; four network and contracting leaders; two utilization management leaders; two community relations and product management leaders and staff members; two chief medical officers; two plan medical directors; and six behavioral health medical directors. Quality improvement team members interviewed included 12 quality improvement strategy or corporate quality directors and staff members. In addition to medical personnel employed in the positions referenced above, to obtain information on beneficiary outreach and management and implementation of quality improvement strategies, we interviewed clinical stakeholders, including nine health plan affiliated providers, four case management team members, and nine care coordinator team members.

Interviews with the health plan stakeholders revealed several factors that health plans perceive as influencing their ability to initiate and engage beneficiaries in SUD treatment. Results from the qualitative analyses are grouped by qualitative research question, and brief deidentified summaries of health plan visits are included in Appendix F.

Qualitative Research Question 1: Which Types of Health Plan Characteristics and Strategies Are Demonstrated by Plans with Higher Performance or Greater Improvement in IET in SUD and OUD Treatment?

Health Plan Governance and Organizational Structure

Interviewees were asked to describe their health plan structure, including leadership organization and governance over behavioral health services and SUD IET strategies. Health plan representatives generally described a multilevel governance approach, including corporate and local oversight of behavioral health care, which included SUD services. National or regional insurance companies operating state Medicaid plans described varying mixtures of centralized, corporate oversight for behavioral health with local execution of procedures and policies regarding behavioral health utilization management, care management, and care coordination strategies. National insurance companies operating with centralized corporate leadership noted that their approach enabled them to streamline decision-making and ensure consistency across their business lines, which included other state Medicaid plans, Medicare, and commercial business lines. However, all of the national and regional insurance companies stressed that some level of local decision-making was critical to implementing behavioral health policies and procedures in ways that respond to local population needs.

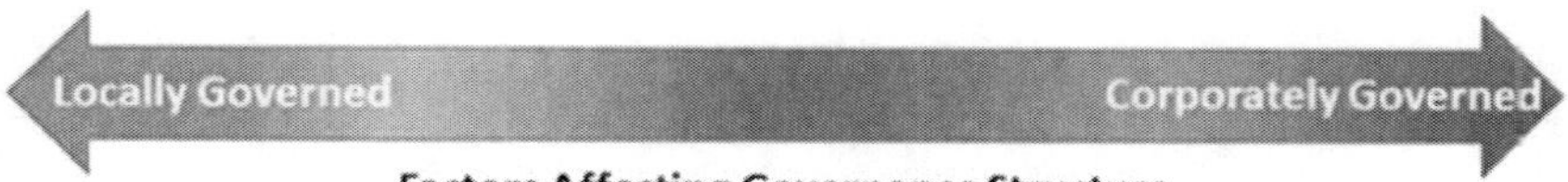

Factors Affecting Governance Structure

- Locus of primary decision-making
- Internal communications strategy
- Processes and structure for quality improvement, monitoring and evaluation
- Policies related to utilization management, care management, care coordination

Figure 9. Spectrum of Governance Structures and Factors Affecting Health Plan Organization.

The extent of health plans' emphasis on local governance represented a spectrum – from having limited local oversight of policy implementation, to equally shared decision-making with the corporate office, to local leadership acting with authority over the majority of health plan operations and corporate executives viewed as consultants for guidance on specific issues (Figure 9). Regional health plans favoring local governance noted that limits on the plan's corporate decision-making were critical to achieving a managed care model that served local population needs. Representatives of these plans described the importance of ensuring local leadership, with state-specific plan presidents, medical directors, and behavioral health directors overseeing locally stationed case management and care coordination teams.

Similarly, plans that serve smaller beneficiary populations or that were not nationally recognized health insurance brands also favored more local control over decision-making and policy implementation efforts. Leadership from locally governed plans described the importance of a "feet-on-the-street" approach, which was supported by the interviews with care managers and others. As such, representatives from locally governed plans frequently described how their organizational structure promoted regular opportunities for communication about beneficiary needs or health services access challenges among plan presidents, medical directors, and staff members directly involved in beneficiary outreach. Health plan representatives described having integrated weekly and monthly rounds with clinicians and oversight staff members to discuss beneficiaries with complex needs or anecdotally observed trends in initiation and engagement success.

The differences in philosophy and approach between the large national plan with more centralized leadership and the regional or small plans with much more local control do not manifest clearly in the plans' relative rates of initiation or engagement on IET or on other behavioral health measures. The state Medicaid plan operated by the large centralized insurer had one of the highest possible rates on initiation but had an engagement rate that was in the 80th percentile. Plans with pronounced local governance had somewhat similar mixtures or had exceptional results on both rates.

Promoting Care Coordination Models and Culture

Interviewees from every health plan described their plan's care model and culture as integral to their success in initiating and engaging beneficiaries in treatment. Care models consistently were described as focused on care coordination. Interviewees emphasized the importance of promoting an understanding of patients' needs for ongoing coordination of physical, mental, behavioral, and substance use-specific services while also managing additional needs such as housing. Having plan-wide care coordination models was described as an actionable way to promote health plans' mission statements and values. Interviewees described their health plan culture – and thus care coordination models – as reflecting a holistic view of member needs, concerned for underserved populations, and focused on collaborative efforts between plan leadership, clinicians, and plan members.

Interviewees commented that their respective health plans sustained and reinforced their care culture and values by tailoring their processes for staff hiring and provider contracting around the plan's mission statements. Most plans described some process for vetting new care coordination staff and clinical providers on the basis of their perceived willingness to approach members' initiation in SUD treatment as a continuous process, rather than an episodic service. Health plan representatives also expressed a desire to hire care managers who were willing to go beyond phone outreach and follow up with members in the community, including conducting house calls, meeting in hospitals or detox facilities, or locating them at community-based recovery support services. Additionally, plan representatives generally described hiring requirements for outreach staff that extended beyond clinical competency and focused on soft skills including communication and demonstrating empathy and patience with members.

Interviewees at high performing plans also described a preference for hiring care managers and care coordinators who were skilled clinicians with master's degrees and a few years of experience in a variety of care coordination roles. Effective care coordinators and outreach workers frequently were described as "trouble shooters" who can identify members' unmet needs. Plan representatives described hiring for a variety of outreach and care coordination roles. Behavioral health and medical care managers frequently are used to conduct face-to-face visits with members, coordinate care plans, and review entitlements. Plans use clinical community specialists and community health workers to conduct community outreach with hard-to-reach members including homeless individuals.

All the health plan representatives described the role of hiring case managers, care coordinators, and community health workers as promoting beneficiaries' use of services included within the plan's benefit array. However, several plans also described these staff members as critical to identifying additional community-based recovery supports for members beyond the plan's covered benefits. Health plans expect these staff members to coordinate external recovery supports in the hope that members would maintain engagement with treatment services longer and become more stable.

Health plan leadership and network contracting staff members described efforts to convey the health plan's mission statement when meeting with new providers. Health plan representatives generally expressed a desire to expand their provider network, but many were concerned about including providers that do not emulate their health plan values. Provider contracting teams described meeting with new providers to reinforce the plans' commitment to continuous engagement with beneficiaries – that repeated successes and failures with SUD treatment initiation are part of the recovery process and providers must continuously engage patients in communication about the benefits of treatment. The goal is to repeatedly reinforce this message so that, if the patient is hearing this on a day when he or she is receptive, the provider will be able to initiate a treatment plan with the patient. Plan representatives described hiring or contracting with providers and staff members who would promote a culture of acceptance among staff and members.

Benefit Array

Health plan representatives described significant differences in their benefit arrays. Medicaid plan representatives consistently described coverage of outpatient and inpatient services, but some stated that they do not reimburse for certain of the intermediate services such as partial hospitalization, and only one reimbursed for limited residential care. Half of the Medicaid plan representatives also described the need for prior authorization before members could engage in several types of SUD treatment services. However, none of the Medicaid plans required beneficiaries to pay for any services out-of-pocket. The representative of the commercial plan interviewed for this study described the plan's benefit array as an "all-you-can-eat buffet" of services for beneficiaries, free of prior authorization or utilization management review. Although the plan covers an expansive continuum of SUD treatment services, members are required to meet their plan deductible prior to having all service costs reimbursed by the plan. Deductibles vary on the basis of individual plans offered through the commercial insurer.

Significant Differences
Health plan representatives described significant differences in their benefit arrays.

Representatives of only two plans described having implemented universal early intervention activities such as SBIRT. One Medicaid plan implemented universal SBIRT to screen for all alcohol and other substance misuse for all beneficiaries aged 12 years and older. One Medicaid plan representative described providers' initial hesitation to conduct SBIRT because of uncertainty about how to talk about substance use and competing priorities during the visit.

The plan representative noted that SBIRT adoption into practice ultimately was driven by a statewide performance measure that put the plan financially at risk for uptake. The commercial plan implements a homegrown SBIRT-like model to screen for risk of alcohol use disorder but does not conduct screening for illicit substances. With the support of its research department, the plan staff developed an alcohol screening form in-house. Initially the commercial plan requested that clinicians conduct brief interventions using evidence-based motivational interviewing techniques. However, clinicians expressed discomfort with the process, and the plan shifted its SBIRT model to require that clinicians provide members with harm reduction advice prior to making a referral to a follow-up visit. To aid in this process, the commercial plan developed a loose script for clinicians to reference when giving advice. The script mirrors the way in which clinicians talk about diabetes care management and being above or below target levels. Clinicians inform plan members about guidelines for safe drinking, and then the clinician and plan member discuss whether the member's drinking behavior is above or below those guidelines. Harm reduction strategies such as reducing the number of daily drinks or binge drinking episodes are discussed with plan members exceeding safe drinking guidelines.

All six plans cover some medically monitored and medically managed detox services, although representatives from half of the plans described requiring either a prior authorization or some other type of access notification when plan members are admitted to these services. One plan in a non-expansion state covers only detox services for pregnant women. All plans cover outpatient treatment services without prior authorization. However, inpatient services, including intensive inpatient and partial hospitalization services, frequently were described as requiring prior authorization from health plans. Representatives from plans requiring some level of notification for any of these services indicated that the condition was not meant to limit or delay access to care but rather was a method of tracking members and identifying individuals in need of case management or care coordination services and follow-up.

Medicaid plan representatives described limitations on their ability to reimburse for residential treatment services because of state Medicaid policy. Four of the five Medicaid plan interview groups said that their state Medicaid agency did not include residential treatment in Medicaid benefits for non-pregnant beneficiaries. The representative from one Medicaid plan with a residential treatment benefit described being able to approve their members' residential services only in 7-day increments and with a total average length of stay of 30-days. Because of the state Medicaid benefit limits on residential services, most plan representatives described having their case managers and care coordinators outreach to community-based programs and grants to help members identify funding for residential treatment. In contrast, the commercial plan representative reported residential services as a covered benefit.

Naltrexone

Representatives from only 1 Medicaid plan and the commercial plan indicated that they include naltrexone in injection form on their formularies. High cost was cited as a barrier for inclusion.

All health plans provide members with coverage of at least two MAT medication options for opioid treatment. All plan representatives reported covering buprenorphine or buprenorphine-naloxone medications as well as methadone. However, multiple plans described a preference for referring members to buprenorphine prescribers over methadone clinics because of plans' ability to coordinate member services with plan-affiliated prescribers rather than having to develop relationships and share records with external methadone clinics. The representative from one Medicaid plan also described a state policy that required beneficiaries to access methadone as a carved-out benefit through another state plan that specifically handled methadone treatment. Although the state recently had allowed its Medicaid managed care plans to coordinate benefits for methadone maintenance, the plan representative indicated that the plan's history with the carve-out model still deters the plan from promoting methadone. Representatives from only one Medicaid plan and the commercial plan indicated that they include naltrexone in injection form on their formularies. Plan representatives frequently cited the high cost of injectable naltrexone as a barrier to including it on their preferred drug lists.

Most plan representatives noted that they did not require prior authorization for MAT. They said that removing prior authorizations was important to ensuring access to necessary SUD treatment. However, one described maintaining prior authorization for all types of MAT. Although the state Medicaid benefit did not require prior authorization, the plan representative noted that it was beneficial to ensuring that the plan was knowledgeable about which beneficiaries were receiving these services. The plan also wanted to ensure that all beneficiaries initiating MAT also were participating in some other SUD treatment service such as one-on-one or group counseling. The plan representatives described their MAT service authorization similarly to how other plan representatives expressed a need for prior authorization on detoxification services. The approval was not meant to serve as an access restraint but to keep the plan informed about which beneficiaries were engaging in SUD treatment services and might require additional care coordination.

Naloxone formulations are included on all the interviewed plan drug formularies. None of the plan representatives described having specific coprescribing practices in place to direct providers to prescribe naloxone to members at risk for overdose. However, most indicated that they would be receptive to covering the cost of naloxone so that a beneficiary's family member could carry the overdose reversal medication in case of emergency. Leadership at three of the interviewed plans said that this topic had been discussed previously in meetings about improving SUD treatment outcomes. Representatives from the commercial plan were more familiar with providing naloxone to family members of beneficiaries at risk for overdose. Plan leadership described a state law that required plans to make the medication available to family members of beneficiaries at the same cost that the plan member would pay. Plan leadership was supportive of the legislation and the plan's ability to promote access to the life-saving medication.

Coverage of recovery support services was sparse among Medicaid plans. In some cases, peer supports are not a covered state benefit and, in at least one instance, the plan did not use peer support even though the state covered it. The commercial plan provides members with access to peer supports as part of their *service buffet* offered at all SUD treatment clinics affiliated with the plan. Their plan members have access to individual and group counseling as well as to educational groups focused on relationship building, anger management, depression, mindfulness, and other holistic recovery supports at the plan-affiliated clinics.

Although most Medicaid plans do not operate their own educational and recovery support groups, they do rely on outreach workers and case managers to identify community-based supports for their beneficiaries. Representatives from all but one Medicaid plan described sending outreach staff into the community to cultivate partnerships with external peer supports, education, and sober living organizations.

Quality Improvement Activities

Health plans engage in SUD treatment-related quality improvement in a variety of ways (Figure 10). Representatives from nationally branded plans and those with greater membership populations report employing large quality improvement teams that include statisticians and leadership to continuously monitor data trends in diagnostics and service use. Representatives from plans with limited resources or those without fully integrated EHRs described focusing on enhancing communication channels between beneficiaries and the plan and between case management teams and plan leadership to identify emerging needs of their covered lives. Almost all plan representatives also spoke about the importance of engaging with their provider population to promote uptake of evidence-based practices relevant to imitation and engagement in SUD treatment.

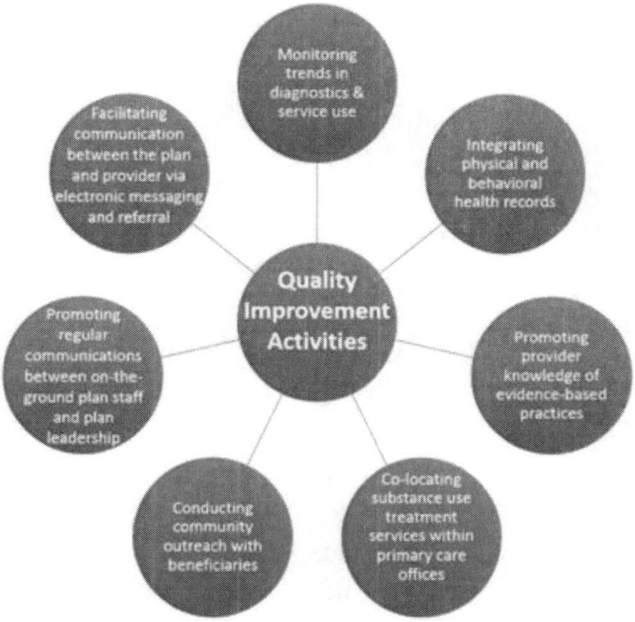
Monitoring trends in diagnostics & service use
Integrating physical and behavioral health records
Promoting provider knowledge of evidence-based practices
Co-locating substance use treatment services within primary care offices
Conducting community outreach with beneficiaries
Promoting regular communications between on-the-ground plan staff and plan leadership
Facilitating communication between the plan and provider via electronic messaging and referral
Quality Improvement Activities

Figure 10. Quality Improvement Activities Used by Health Plans.

Health plans struggle overall to achieve full integration of their electronic medical records. However, multiple plan leadership groups reported investing significant resources in developing fully integrated physical and behavioral health records. Integrated records were described as a cutting-edge way for plans to more deeply understand their membership needs. Integrated health records allow health plan quality improvement teams to measure the frequency of acute care services or diagnostic risk factors for SUDs in their population. Plan representatives generally noted confidence in their ability to identify members with the most severe health needs. However, plan interviewees described investing in data analytics to identify members with moderate health risks and proactively outreach these individuals with additional supports. For example, one plan is conducting a monthly analysis of its pharmacy data to identify any members who billed for three or more narcotic prescriptions, dispensed by three or more pharmacies, with prescriptions written by three or more prescribers. The plan interviewee said that this monthly report generates a surprisingly long list of beneficiaries, including a significant portion who do not have any SUD or mental health diagnosis in their medical record. The plan then shares their monthly report with its care coordination team to identify next steps for member outreach.

Plan interviewees also described using integrated EHRs to track members' progression from a positive identification for substance use risk through treatment initiation and engagement over time. The commercial plan integrated a universal alcohol SBIRT screening form into their medical record. Any members who screen positive for risky alcohol use are flagged for follow-up. The plan generates a daily report of all members who are identified as having risky alcohol use and monitors those individuals for receipt of treatment referral and completion of follow-up appointments. A monthly report is generated for each plan-affiliated provider practice to identify members with a positive alcohol screen, the date of their positive screen, whether a referral was made, whether a follow-up appointment and assessment were scheduled and completed, whether the member has since initiated any SUD treatment services, and the name of the member's PCP. The plan implemented provider change leaders in each affiliated practice to support their effort. Change leaders are selected by the physicians within the local practice group and are responsible for reviewing the monthly reports with all physicians in their group. Change leaders are helping this plan bridge its advanced data analytic capabilities with more traditional quality improvement focused communication strategies.

All interviewed health plan representatives described open communication within the plan and between the plan and its membership as key to achieving improvements in SUD treatment. Communication strategies included using secure electronic messaging services to maintain real-time communication with providers concerning high-risk beneficiaries, including those with a newly diagnosed SUD. Similar to the intent of daily or monthly reports that identify members in need of follow-up services, plans are using secure messaging systems to send providers reminders to conduct follow-up calls and send outreach letters. Interviewees also described these systems as critical ways for providers to reach out to the plan directly, indicating whether the provider thinks that a plan member could benefit from care coordination or outreach efforts orchestrated by the plan. Providers can essentially "refer" a plan member for care coordination services to be provided by their health plan. Health plan care coordinators or outreach workers then phone the member to discuss his or her care needs. Outreach teams are trained on effective communication techniques to encourage members to engage in treatment.

Co-Locating Services

Representatives from only 1 Medicaid plan and the commercial plan indicated that they include naltrexone in injection form on their formularies. High cost was cited as a barrier for inclusion. One plan stated that, prior to co-locating its SUD treatment counselors in primary care settings, only approximately 25% of the members they identified as in need of treatment actually initiated services.

Ensuring regular opportunities for open communication between care coordinators, outreach workers, case managers, and plan leadership including behavioral health medical directors were cited frequently as essential to improving treatment initiation and engagement. Every interviewed plan described some form of regularly scheduled in-person or conference call meeting for health plan staff members to discuss general treatment initiation challenges or to focus on strategies to improve outcomes for individual members with complex needs. As previously noted, many interviewees considered these regular meetings a critical way to keep plan governance leadership informed of membership needs. Interviewees from multiple plans described several occasions in which meetings between case managers and plan leadership resulted in the plan providing additional support to meet specific member needs. For example, interviewees described using plan funds to cover non-reimbursable costs for transportation or authorizing additional hospitalization days for members who otherwise would be discharged into unsafe living arrangements.

Overall, health plan interviewees expressed a substantial interest in maintaining communication between physical health and behavioral health providers. Primary care provider visits are seen as plans' first opportunity to identify the unmet behavioral health needs of their membership population.

Several plans described the importance of co-locating primary care and SUD treatment services as a way to improve treatment initiation. Interviewees described co-locating behavioral health counselors in primary care practices as critical to treatment initiation for patients who otherwise would not attend services provided in a behavioral health facility. One plan anecdotally described that, prior to co-locating its SUD treatment counselors in primary care settings, only approximately 25 percent of the members they identified as in need of treatment actually initiated services. Interviewees also use co-location as a strategy to overcome patient stigma around attending treatment services. The plan estimates that its SUD follow-up rate is now 80 percent. Embedding SUD counselors in primary care practices also was seen as improving communication between different specialty providers, which facilitated outreach efforts to plan members. If a member has disengaged from SUD treatment but attends a primary care or other medical appointment, the embedded SUD counselor can do a quick face-to-face visit to motivate that member to re-engage in services.

Many of the health plan representatives described plans to continue expanding efforts to co-locate services as a way to facilitate initiation in SUD treatment. For example, members with mental health needs frequently attend group sessions, which gives them little time to attend one-on-one or group SUD sessions. Co-locating these sessions in the same facility or developing more co-occurring group sessions for mental health and SUD issues would help more members initiate treatment for their SUD diagnosis. Plan providers described co-location as a critical part of their success in treating patients with SUDs.

Finally, health plans described provider education efforts as an essential piece of their quality improvement strategies. One health plan, however, expressed concern about burdening providers who must work with multiple insurers and indicated a disinclination to target education or initiatives directly at providers, but this plan did not hesitate to engage in quality improvement targeted at beneficiaries. Other plans were conscientious about not wanting to inundate providers with too much information but aimed to carefully disseminate information about targeted best practices in SUD treatment. Interviewees described developing monthly webinars, newsletters, and health plan meetings to promote understanding of evidence-based practices with providers. Interviewees described these efforts as a way to motivate providers while encouraging their accountability for quality health outcomes in the membership population.

Health plans reported investing significant resources in their quality improvement activities including developing new staff positions to support activities, investing in software to develop their data analytic capabilities, and establishing secure communications with beneficiaries and providers. Representatives from two of the Medicaid plans reported focusing their time and financial investments on initiatives that targeted activities related to service and quality measures for which they were financially at risk under the state Medicaid plan. These plans are motivated to maximize their returns on those metrics. Although many of the Medicaid plans are part of value-based purchasing at the state level, at the time of interview the majority of plans included in this study were not engaging in value-based payment arrangements with providers related to substance use metrics. At least two changes that are anticipated in the near future would involve providers in shared savings arrangements. However, all plans expressed an interest in closely managing their SUD population in an effort to manage overall costs. Generally, plan representatives expressed a concern that poorly managed SUDs would result in higher overall costs incurred at the emergency department or other ambulatory care service providers.

Qualitative Research Question 2: What Other Factors (e.g., Patient, Setting, Provider, State, and Local Market Characteristics) Do Health Plans Identify as Affecting Rates of Initiation and Engagement in SUD and OUD Treatment?

Health plan interviewees described four key external factors they felt affected health plans' effectiveness at initiating and engaging members in SUD treatment services:

1) Federal and state policies – specifically federal privacy and Medicaid-specific policies— were identified as major factors affecting health plans' ability to provide comprehensive services to meet membership needs.
2) Stigma around SUD and mental health treatment was cited repeatedly as a major barrier to treatment initiatives.
3) Plan member attitudes toward treatment and receiving support from their health plan were cited as substantially affecting treatment uptake.
4) All health plan representatives cited a general concern over network adequacy for SUD treatment services as both a current concern and a major barrier to future access to treatment.

Policy Factors

Health plans described federal confidentiality requirements of the 42 Code of Federal Regulations (CFR) Part 2 as specifically challenging to coordinating care for members admitted to detox and other inpatient facilities. 42 CFR Part 2 was established to restrict the disclosure of medical records describing an individual's diagnosis with an SUD or receipt of SUD treatment. The regulation requires individuals to provide consent to share any records pertaining to services received for SUD treatment. Several health plan representatives described detox facilities' understanding of the release of information requirements for 42 CFR Part 2 as overly burdensome to their ability to outreach to members prior to discharge and not reflective of the actual regulation requirements. Two plans addressed the recent amendments to the regulation and indicated that the amendments did not effectively address the needs of health plans to be able to coordinate care for their members. One interviewee characterized the recent amendment to the regulation as having "wasted an opportunity."

Shortages of Residential Placements

One barrier to obtaining residential treatment for Medicaid health plan members is the prohibition against Medicaid reimbursement in so-called IMDs with more than 15 beds. This means that many Medicaid health plans do not reimburse for residential services. States, however, are increasingly seeking Section 1115 waivers to allow such reimbursement under their state Medicaid plans. Some health plans also seek residential placements with fewer than 16 beds so that reimbursement can be obtained. Despite these efforts, significant shortages of residential beds are reported, sometimes resulting in health plan members leaving detoxification and re-entering the community prematurely.

Multiple health plan stakeholders described learning of beneficiary detox admissions only after the beneficiary had been discharged from the facility. Case managers expressed frustration about being unable to engage in predischarge planning or identify new contact information on the plan members prior to their discharge. Case managers at one of the health plans described spending a significant amount of time working to improve their relationship with local detox facilities. The case managers are hoping that their positive relationships with the detox facilities will encourage facility staff to reach out to them, within the confines of 42 CFR Part 2, when their plan beneficiaries are admitted for detox services.

Each of the five Medicaid plan representatives interviewed identified policies emanating from their state Medicaid agency as factors limiting their ability to initiate and engage members in SUD treatment. Most of the Medicaid plans viewed restrictions on the types of services included in the state Medicaid benefit array as a substantial barrier. These included consistent restrictions on reimbursement for residential care given the federal prohibition on reimbursement for IMDs. Only one plan representative described the state service benefit as providing the full continuum of SUD treatment services, but with restricted ability to reimburse for residential treatment. Health plan representatives expressed a desire to cover additional treatment services not reimbursable by the state but ultimately noted that doing so was beyond their financial capability. Medicaid plan representatives described operating under a tight budget without sufficient funds to provide recovery supports outside of the state benefit.

State Medicaid policies that allow beneficiaries to frequently switch plans also were identified as negatively affecting health plans' ability to coordinate services. Many of the Medicaid plans interviewed had authority from the state to place beneficiaries in pharmacy or prescriber lock-in programs. Plan representatives described using these programs when beneficiaries were identified as receiving several prescriptions for controlled substances such as opioid analgesics from multiple prescribers or pharmacies. A few Medicaid plan representatives described placing beneficiaries in lock-in programs to monitor their prescription use while conducting outreach and case management efforts, only to have the beneficiary switch to another Medicaid plan mid-year. Some health plans reported frequent movement of Medicaid beneficiaries across state plans throughout a single enrollment year. One plan noted that the state Medicaid agency had further restricted movement between plans to control "plan shopping" to evade pharmacy and provider lock-ins.

Battling Stigma

Health plans reported investing time in supporting community education about SUDs and the positive impact of treatment as ways to reduce stigma both in the community at large and in the minds of individuals who might need treatment.

Stigma

Health plan representatives commented on the ways in which stigma around SUDs and treatment hindered their ability to effectively initiate and engage members in treatment services. Health plans are cognizant of how community stigma toward SUD issues prevents individuals from identifying a personal need for care and reaching out for support. One interviewee who is actively working to cultivate working relationships between her health plan and local community organizations described the isolating effect of stigma. Although families experiencing a cancer diagnosis are supported by the community at large, families dealing with an SUD are not comforted in the same way. Other interviewees echoed this sentiment and described how neighborhood stigma can prevent their plan members from wanting to participate in recovery supports that do exist in their community. Health plans reported investing time in supporting community education about SUDs and the positive impact of treatment as ways to reduce stigma both in the community at large and in the minds of individuals who might need treatment. One plan also invested in remodeling its SUD treatment clinics to make them blend into the local neighborhood. The clinics do not include any signage identifying them as treatment facilities for SUDs or mental health conditions – rather their facades and waiting rooms are designed as non-specific medical practices.

Health plan representatives also described investing resources in reducing provider stigma around SUDs. Interviewees noted that providers often hesitated to conduct substance use risk screenings because they had not received adequate addictions training in medical school and were uncertain about how to talk to their patients about such issues. One of the interviewed health plans is hoping to improve provider-member conversations about SUD issues by training their members in self-advocacy. The plan sponsored an education class for members to learn about self-efficacy and communications strategies for addressing difficult topics including substance use and unmet care needs.

Health plan representatives also said that, although provider stigma related to treating members with an SUD has improved, many providers still were hesitant to take on new patients, especially those with Medicaid benefits. Plan representatives described conversations with providers expressing concern about Medicaid beneficiaries being disruptive in waiting rooms and burglarizing their practices for prescription drugs.

Members' Competing Needs and Attitudes toward Treatment

Interviewees described plan members' competing priorities including housing, child care, and accessing treatment for comorbid physical and behavioral health conditions as factors affecting successful initiation or continued engagement in substance use treatment services. Beneficiaries who are homeless or transient were identified as challenging to engage because they do not have stable addresses or phone numbers, which would facilitate outreach efforts. Most of the health plan representatives reported employing case managers and outreach workers based in the local community as a way to engage with community supports that their members might access.

Health plans also described efforts to provide members with transportation to follow-up appointments as a means of ensuring attendance. Health plans reported providing bus passes, reimbursing taxi costs, and providing gas cards to help individuals with limited finances overcome transportation barriers. Despite being able to offer these supports, case managers indicated that beneficiaries' attendance at follow-up appointments still was impeded by competing demands. For example, one plan representative explained that although members were provided a transportation benefit to get to their appointments, the state restricted children from accompanying members in the vehicle with them. Thus, to make their SUD appointment, beneficiaries with transportation and child care needs face the challenge of securing alternative transportation or a babysitter. Interviewed plan case managers said that most beneficiaries in this predicament simply do not attend treatment.

Health plan interviewees acknowledged that many of their beneficiaries with an SUD also have co-occurring medical and/or other health conditions that hinder their ability to attend SUD appointments or achieve medication adherence. Health plans responded by encouraging their care managers and outreach workers to meet members where they are and to prioritize member-identified needs. Health plan interviewees noted that implementing this approach resulted in the plan becoming aware of a member's need for SUD treatment, but it did not push the member to immediately engage in those services. Health plans focusing on this patient-centered approach noted that it was a strategy for keeping the door open to future SUD treatment.

Interviews also revealed that health plans are deeply concerned about being seen as a trustworthy resource to their members. Several health plans described member attitudes toward SUD treatment and health systems in general as a significant factor affecting their decision to initiate treatment. Health plan representatives noted that members often viewed the plan as an extension of untrustworthy state or other health care systems that they had encountered in the past. As a result, members were reluctant to respond to health plan outreach efforts. In response, these health plans are invested in developing positive relationships with community-based organizations that their members know. For example, one health plan representative described having the plan's outreach workers frequent community centers and treatment facilities that its members attend. Over time, the outreach workers became more familiar to both the community organizations and the plan members who frequent those centers. Integrating plan outreach workers in the community enabled the plan members to begin trusting the outreach workers and the health plan. Plan members now are more responsive to outreach efforts and care coordination from the health plan.

Requirements for Access beyond Network Adequacy

All of the health plans described specific network adequacy requirements including limits on the mileage and travel time for beneficiaries to access treatment providers. Although each of the health plans are meeting these requirements set out by the state Medicaid agency and their governance boards, interviewees repeatedly described having additional network needs. Interviewees expressed concern over the growing need for treatment coinciding with decreases in the number of medical doctors specializing in SUD treatment. Health plan representatives focused most frequently, however, on how limited access to Drug

Addiction Treatment Act of 2000 (DATA 2000)-waivered buprenorphine prescribers and residential treatment beds serve as barriers to meeting the treatment needs of their plan members.

Network Adequacy Issues

Growing need for treatment coincides with:

- Decreases in the number of providers specializing in SUD treatment.
- Limited access to buprenorphine prescribers.
- Providers who do not accept Medicaid beneficiaries.
- Lack of residential beds.
- Low reimbursement rates that limit plans' abilities to expand network adequacy for necessary services.

Health plan representatives described actively working on expanding their MAT provider networks. One health plan representative reported having its provider relations team conduct monthly outreach to assess which buprenorphine prescribers are accepting new patients. Representatives from this plan indicated that their efforts have not been successful in expanding their network adequacy for MAT. They consistently hear that providers do not have openings for their members; however, they are continuing to conduct monthly updates in case prescribers expand their practices. Other Medicaid plan representatives echoed this experience, noting that they find it hard to identify DATA 2000-waivered physicians willing to treat Medicaid beneficiaries. Interviewees said that prescribers would not to take on Medicaid beneficiaries because of preconceived notions about treating that population or because they were accepting cash only for office visit services.

Interviewees from each of the health plans were quick to identify specific challenges in contracting with sufficient buprenorphine prescribers to expand their treatment capacity. The amount of time spent on documenting buprenorphine treatment to meet DEA requirements was identified as a significant barrier for prescribers. One of the health plans is using grant funding to hire a Certified Alcohol and Drug Abuse Counselor to support a few of the local health plan-affiliated prescribers in multiple aspects of MAT provision, including meeting DEA documentation requirements. The counselor conducts educational consultations with the plan members about buprenorphine treatment, obtains informed consent, and schedules buprenorphine induction. All patient follow-up appointments take place with the counselor and the prescribing physician. Other health plan representatives described a desire to support prescribers in this way but reported lacking funds to pay for this support.

Additionally, health plans are concerned about the lack of beds available to their beneficiaries needing residential treatment facilities. Interviewees at the plan leadership and member outreach levels expressed concern over the lack of residential treatment facilities to which they could send their beneficiaries following discharge from detox services. Interviewees felt that, without residential treatment available to their members, they were watching them get discharged from detox only to relapse in the community without the appropriate level of care to support them.

Low reimbursement rates for both MAT and residential treatment were identified as significant factors limiting plans' ability to expand network adequacy for necessary services and ultimately to ensure access to care for plan beneficiaries. Medicaid plan representatives expressed an inability to contract with providers at reimbursement rates beyond the state rate. Medicaid plans expressed concern that providers withhold open spots from Medicaid beneficiaries to receive greater reimbursement rates from commercial plan members and individuals paying out-of-pocket. Leadership from the commercial plan expressed similar concern over the low rates that Medicaid plans can offer providers. Members of commercial plan leadership said that they are reluctant to reimburse residential treatment providers at rates substantially higher than those set by the state Medicaid agency. Previously the plan had set a higher reimbursement rate for residential providers, but in doing so they priced out the state Medicaid plans. Members of commercial plan leadership also reported reducing their reimbursement rates to help maintain access for Medicaid beneficiaries.

Low Reimbursement
Low reimbursement was identified as a significant factor limiting plans' ability to expand network adequacy for necessary services.

The Medicaid plans do contract on an ad hoc basis with out-of-network providers to fill gaps in access. Payment is negotiated, and most of the Medicaid plans pay the same rate as they do for in-network providers. One plan paid less to provide an incentive to draw providers into the network. One paid more but did not want it widely known. Another plan representative indicated that paying more than a small amount above the state-established rate was burdensome because they would be required to justify doing so to the state.

Qualitative Research Question 3: What Do Health Plan Representatives Believe Are Significant Barriers and Facilitators to Initiating and Engaging Beneficiaries in SUD Treatment?

Overall, health plan representatives did not feel that challenges to initiating members in care differed from the challenges to continued engagement in care. Plan representatives generally noted that any barriers to encouraging members to initiate care were the same barriers that made it easy for members to disengage after a few visits. In response, health plan representatives described identifying and developing facilitation strategies that applied to getting members to both initiate and continuously engage in care.

Key barriers identified by plans relate to community stigma toward SUD and treatment, providers' lack of addiction training and comfort treating individuals with an SUD, plan members' readiness for behavioral change, and service limitations of health plan benefit arrays. Because many of these findings already have been summarized in response to qualitative research Questions 1 and 2, the following section highlights key barriers and their associated facilitators.

Barrier

Community stigma toward SUDs and behavioral health treatment prevents members from initiating and remaining engaged in treatment.

Facilitator

Health plans are focusing on integrating primary care and substance use treatment.

Health plan representatives described substance use-related stigma as communities' rejection and alienation of individuals with an SUD. Interviewees said that communities do not regularly engage in conversations about substance use so it becomes a taboo subject when a community member has an identified need for SUD treatment. Interviewees described stigma around substance use as one of the most significant barriers to encouraging members to initiate and remain engaged in treatment. Health plan representatives identified substance use-related stigma as greater and more isolating than stigma around mental health conditions. Although interviewees noted that alcohol use disorder was less stigmatized than illicit SUD involving heroin or opioid analgesics, they identified overcoming stigma as a challenge to bringing beneficiaries into treatment.

Health plan representatives frequently described considering substance use-related stigma when developing strategies to successfully initiate beneficiaries in treatment. Most commonly, they focused efforts on co-locating SUD treatment services with primary care. Health plan interviewees identified member concerns about attending SUD-specific treatment facilities.

Members did not want to be seen entering these facilities or have medical records specifically list the name of an SUD treatment facility. Interviewees noted that these concerns were particularly troubling for individuals who have not accepted their diagnosis, because they were more likely to perceive SUD treatment facilities as places for individuals with more severe treatment needs. Co-locating SUD treatment services within primary care and other physical health practices encouraged members to attend appointments in a familiar environment without the stigma of being identified as a behavioral health patient.

Warm Hand-Offs

Providers were more comfortable having conversations about substance use risk behavior and treatment initiation with members knowing that they could perform a warm hand-off with the co-located counselor down the hall.

Specifically, most health plan representatives identified embedding SUD treatment counselors within primary care offices as their greatest facilitator to overcoming the beneficiaries' stigma around engaging in treatment. Interviewees said that providers were more comfortable having conversations about substance use risk behavior and treatment initiation with members knowing that they could perform a warm hand-off with the co-located counselor down the hall. Counselors were seen as being able to step in to talk to newly diagnosed members or members with risky behavior about the benefit of initiating some type of treatment. Interviewees also described how embedding counselors improved trust and communication between physical health and SUD treatment providers. Simply having these individuals in the same facility promoted regular conversations about integration and care coordination planning to support members' holistic needs. Interviewees described this integration as key to engaging in routine check-ins with members who are reluctant to initiate treatment or become disengaged over time. Primary care providers are able to repeatedly advise at-risk members about treatment and invite the counselor into the exam room to talk with members about their specific reluctance to initiating treatment. Similarly, co-located substance use counselors can check on members who come in for physical health appointments and make a subsequent effort to engage them in care.

Health plan interviewees described some initial pushback from providers regarding embedding SUD treatment counselors and other integration activities. Some providers told the health plan they felt that the behavioral health counselors were monitoring or infringing on their practice. Health plans responded by having plan leadership reach out to convince providers of the potential benefits of primary and substance use care integration.

Barrier

Providers lack sufficient training in addictions medicine to effectively initiate members in treatment.

Facilitator

Health plans are routinely engaging providers in education opportunities to promote evidence-based practices with substance use treatment.

Health plan interviewees identified primary care providers' lack of addictions training as a critical barrier to identifying risky substance use behavior in members as well as a barrier to encouraging members to initiate and engage in treatment. Interviewees described providers as generally reluctant to conduct screening for risky substance use. Interviewees said that providers reported not feeling comfortable asking the screening questions or knowing how to advise individuals who screened positive. Plan representatives acknowledged that early intervention activities were difficult for providers because substance use risk screening and motivational interviewing techniques were not adequately covered in medical school training.

As a result, health plan interviewees described developing a variety of educational opportunities directed at enhancing providers' knowledge of best practices for substance use screening and treatment.

Health plans that require providers to conduct universal SBIRT with plan members reported developing training modules specific to using the screening tool and to conducting the brief intervention component for members with an identified risk. One plan representative reported holding provider training sessions on how to conduct motivational interviews with members.

Providers practiced motivational interviewing techniques in person to develop confidence with the early intervention practice. Another plan reported abandoning the traditional motivational interviewing component of SBIRT in favor of having providers simply offer advice about reducing substance use. After providers reported feeling unsuccessful with the original motivational interviewing requirement, local plan leadership provided them with risk reduction talking points that mimic how providers counsel diabetic patients about glucose levels.

Members are advised on the safe range of alcohol consumption and how much they would need to reduce consumption to be considered within safe medical guidelines.

Health plan representatives also reported developing electronic referral, messaging, and reporting tools to facilitate providers' efforts to initiate and engage beneficiaries in treatment. Multiple health plans invested in creating provider portals or other electronic systems to promote effortless communication between the provider and the health plan. Such systems are enabling providers to refer plan members to care coordination services and follow-up care with a single click. When this referral is made, health plans are alerted to the request in real-time and begin conducting outreach with the plan member. Health plan representatives said that they were motivated to create these tools to partially remove the burden of treatment initiation from primary care providers. Instead, the plan can outreach members directly to encourage treatment uptake.

Half of the health plan representatives interviewed also described generating provider reports on the number of members with an identified SUD and their follow-up treatment status.

Interviewees noted that plan staff meet one-on-one with providers to discuss their performance and identify next steps for engaging members in treatment. Similarly, health plans are developing regularly scheduled meetings with providers to discuss best practices in SUD treatment. Plan interviewees described these in-person and webinar meetings as opportunities to inform providers about practices that close the gap between SUD diagnosis and treatment initiation. Meetings highlight the importance of referring members for care coordination and case management. Meetings also highlight best practices regarding MAT and ASAM criteria regarding level of care and care transitions. Health plans also are promoting materials developed by SAMHSA to augment provider knowledge around evidence-based practices in SUD treatment. Two of the health plans also reported partnering with local subject matter experts and university researchers to promote providers' understanding of the local populations' needs and attitudes toward SUD treatment.

Overall, health plan representatives noted that their many efforts to educate providers about substance use issues and treatment processes are helping them engage members in treatment. Most interviewees described wanting to serve as a support for providers and viewed the health plan and providers as part of the same team trying to bring members into care. Health plans are promoting this team sentiment by carefully scripting the way that they approach education with providers. Interviewees said that they were cognizant of not wanting to come off as telling physicians how to operate, but they want providers to see best practices and electronic systems as valuable tools for their patients.

Barrier

Members are not ready to abstain from substance use or other related risk behaviors, which results in an unwillingness to initiate traditional SUD treatment.

Facilitator

Health plans are promoting harm reduction techniques and "no wrong door" and "no wrong time" approaches to engage members in conversations about substance use.

Health plan interviewees identified beneficiaries' readiness to abstain from substance use as a significant factor affecting their ability to initiate or sustain engagement in treatment programs.

They described treatment programs and care management as historically focused on an abstinence-only approach with sobriety as a key requirement for continued engagement. Interviewees generally agreed that promoting abstinence-only treatment environments did not facilitate initiating members in treatment. As a result, health plan interviewees reported gradually shifting their approach to promoting harm reduction environments as well as abstinence programs. Representatives from several plans identified this shift to harm reduction as a significant facilitator for both initiating members in treatment and maintaining long-term engagement.

When Health Plan Members Do Not Feel Ready for Treatment

Health plans are more frequently promoting harm reduction techniques and "no wrong door" and "no wrong time" approaches to engage members in conversations about substance use.

Health plan representatives reported offering a variety of harm reduction initiatives to members. One plan began sponsoring group sessions that promote conversations between members who are reducing their use but have not fully quit. The plan representative noted that these groups have been useful for bringing more people into service who did not previously self-identify as needing treatment. The harm reduction groups were described as a place for members to begin thinking about what treatment would mean for them and what healthful behaviors are helpful to them in achieving their personal goals. Health plan representatives also described having care managers and outreach workers identify community-based harm reduction programs for members to participate in as a first step to reducing risky behavior.

Plans described harm reduction strategies as an extension of their intent to promote patient-centered care coordination and a "no wrong door" approach to SUD treatment. Health plan representatives described their no wrong door approach as enabling members to engage in any kind of treatment services, whether it be physical or behavioral health-focused, and then building a trusting relationship with the member to support initiation and engagement in SUD treatment. In developing an ongoing relationship with members, health plan interviewees noted that they can engage beneficiaries in treatment as soon as members express an interest. Thus, the no wrong door perspective also is facilitating a "no wrong time" approach to getting members into SUD treatment.

Discussions around the no wrong door approach focused on asking members about their priorities and health goals. Health plan representatives acknowledged that this approach was more easily promoted through their own care management and care coordination staff than through their contracted providers. The challenge with adopting this approach, according to interviewees, is that it requires a culture change from the way SUD treatment is traditionally viewed. Health plans are using their staff to promote a patient-centered philosophy rather than a program-centric approach.

Barrier

Health plan benefit arrays do not sufficiently cover the continuum of SUD treatment; this limits members' ability to initiate treatment or continue engaging in services that appropriately support their recovery needs.

Facilitator

Health plans are investing in staff that support members' access to community-based recovery supports and perform outreach to support treatment initiation and engagement.

One of the most significant themes identified in the health plan interviews is how health plans are focused on promoting a care coordination model that is based in mission statements about individualized and patient-centered care. This approach enables health plans to stretch beyond their stewardship of plan benefits to support beneficiaries with care management and outreach and to facilitate engagement in community-based recovery supports.

Plan-employed care managers, care coordinators, community health workers, and other outreach workers were identified as critical to successfully initiating and engaging members in treatment. Health plan interviewees repeatedly acknowledged that their ability to bring members into SUD treatment was contingent on their understanding that members have needs beyond traditional health services. Health plans are staffing their care management, coordination, and outreach teams with clinicians who are experienced and licensed and have a master's degree. Health plans expect these clinicians to conduct face-to-face visits as well as telephonic outreach with members wherever they are in the community. When plans learn of member admissions to detox or other inpatient facilities, these clinicians are expected to conduct immediate outreach with the member. Clinicians in these roles described reaching out to members to participate in discharge planning and care transitions and to coordinate community-based treatment postdischarge. Interviewees reported sharing their care plans with members' providers to facilitate ongoing treatment efforts and to integrate members' physical and behavioral health care.

Interviewees also reported a consistent expectation from their health plans to understand members' holistic needs across substance use, mental health, physical health, and necessities such as housing and food. Interviewees consistently described clinicians in these roles as "going above and beyond" for health plan members. But health plan representatives repeatedly described this level of member outreach as the primary facilitator of getting members to the initial SUD treatment visit and ensuring that they continued engaging long-term. Health plan interviewees noted that focusing on their members' individual needs enables their plans to identify key moments when members are receptive to treatment.

Community Partnerships

Interviewees reported establishing relationships with community-based peer support services, educational and employment support agencies, sober housing agencies, and other tenancy support organizations.

Additionally, interviewees at all five Medicaid plans identified limits on their covered services as restricting access to necessary treatment and recovery supports. As previously discussed, health plan representatives expressed frustration about not always being able to link their beneficiaries to partial hospitalization and residential treatment. Some of the Medicaid plans also were unable to reimburse for peer support services, which their representatives unanimously felt would facilitate their members' engagement in recovery.

Because of service limits within their own benefits, representatives from all five Medicaid plans reported cultivating community partnerships to expand their access to recovery supports across systems. Although they reported being unable to reimburse for these services directly, they can refer members to the services and help identify grant or donation funding for members when necessary. Interviewees reported establishing relationships with community-based peer support services, educational and employment support agencies, sober housing agencies, and other tenancy support organizations.

Care managers, care coordinators, community health workers, and other plan-employed outreach workers are expected to cultivate these community relationships to increase supports available to members. Health plan leadership frequently described these non-reimbursable services as key to promoting stability in members' lives and thus promoting their continued engagement in SUD treatment. Representatives from half of the plans interviewed reported encouraging their staff members to inform leadership about the success of these community partnerships. They described efforts to track and report on member progress as a means of producing evidence that might support possible inclusion of these services in the plan benefit array in the future.

Facilitators and Barriers to Measurement for HEDIS IET

The primary aims of the qualitative interviews and analyses were focused on identifying characteristics, strategies, and other factors that affect the ability of successful health plans to initiate and engagement members in care. However, several health plans also wanted to discuss ways in which they view the criteria of the HEDIS IET measure as affecting their measured success in initiating or engaging members in treatment. The following themes are drawn from brief conversations with health plans around the structure or calculation of the HEDIS IET measures.

Health plan representatives expressed concern about the timeline by which the IET measure requires them to meet the initiation and engagement phases of the measure. The initiation phase requires individuals to receive inpatient or outpatient treatment within 14 days of an initial SUD diagnosis. Health plans have a total of 30 days from the member's first visit in which to complete two additional treatment visits and achieve engagement. Health plan representatives indicated that they often did not receive claims data on their members within those time frames, and thus they were unable to ensure that members receiving an initial diagnosis completed initial and follow-up visits in time to count toward the measure. Plan representatives noted that if they failed to receive timely notice of a member's initial detox admission, they likely would fail both the initiation and engagement phases of the measure.

Health plans also commented on the measure's requirement that the initial diagnosis and initial outpatient or inpatient visit occur with different providers if they are completed on the same day. Representatives from two of the health plans commented that they had previously encouraged diagnosing providers to walk members into follow-up appointments with different providers in order to meet the initiation phase. One reported having financially incented providers to conduct this warm hand-off. Health plans enjoyed the option to count same-day appointments toward the measure requirements and expressed concern over the criteria being changed to require that all visits occur on different dates.

Finally, one health plan representative noted that the measurement criteria used for commercial and Medicaid beneficiaries should differ. Plan representatives described how general sociodemographic differences between commercial and Medicaid beneficiaries should alter the expectations for treatment initiation and engagement timelines. The health plan interviewees specifically highlighted challenges in locating Medicaid beneficiaries who are homeless or otherwise hard to reach. Plan interviewees noted that the timeline for meeting the initiation and engagement phases of the measure should be extended for Medicaid populations.

SYNTHESIS OF FINDINGS AND STUDY IMPLICATIONS

The opioid crisis has worsened a pre-existing failure to adequately provide SUD treatment to many in the United States who desperately need it. Many people in need of treatment do not attempt to access it, and many who try find access difficult or impossible. As shown in the section of this chapter on Health Plan Trends for the IET Measure, evidence for this worsening crisis may be found in health plan data from across the country, which show declining rates of initiation and engagement in SUD treatment between 2005 and 2014.

To identify factors associated with successful treatment initiation and engagement, including health plan strategies that may increase rates of involvement in treatment, this study looked at models of care, reimbursement, interventions, and best practices that higher-performing health plans use to improve initiation and subsequent engagement in SUD and OUD treatment. We also examined market, provider, and beneficiary factors that affect plan performance in that area.

Our primary focus was to understand how health plans successfully get beneficiaries into SUD treatment and keep them there. For convenience, both in developing quantitative analyses and in identifying health plans to approach and interview, study researchers relied on the HEDIS IET measure. Our real interest, however, lies not in *initiation* and *engagement* as defined by that measure, but in initiation and sustained participation in treatment for as long as the individual patient may require. The IET measure is a tool that got researchers to the point of being able to examine factors that influence initiation and engagement more broadly defined.

Our quantitative analyses linking beneficiary, plan, and market characteristics to commercial health plans, as well as subsequent semi-structured interviews with high performing plans, elucidated key influences identified in the theoretical model (previously described in Figure 1), which, in turn, derived from the existing literature reviewed as part of the environmental scan.

Individual Influences on SUD Treatment Participation

Published literature identifies several individual-level influences on SUD treatment participation. These include individual beliefs and attitudes such as stigma, individual demographic characteristics that may be associated with higher or lower rates of treatment involvement, the nature of a person's substance use (e.g., injection vs. ingested), the person's past experience of SUD treatment, the presence of co-occurring mental health conditions, and level of patient activation. Individual influences most often revealed as affecting initiation and engagement in this study include the individual's sex, competing needs, co-occurring conditions, stigma, and treatment readiness. Successful plans have implemented initiatives designed to address these variables.

Most characteristics that fall within the category of individual influences on initiation and engagement could not be analyzed in the quantitative analyses, but multivariate regressions did show that plans with more female beneficiaries were less likely to perform well on the measure of engagement in SUD treatment and OUD treatment. This finding is consistent with results in the existing literature [7, 8, 9, 10]. Interviews confirmed that health plans have found it harder to engage females than to engage males and indicate that this difference often may result from competing needs, including child care and transportation, that interfere with access to SUD treatment. A woman also may fear loss of custody if she is pregnant or a mother and acknowledges having an SUD and seeks treatment. Approaches that some plans have taken to address the problem of competing needs include the provision of child care to facilitate treatment for mothers and the establishment of a woman's center that specifically addresses pregnant women's treatment needs. As addressed in the results, however, efforts to address these competing needs that are more commonly experienced by females have met with mixed success but have been shown to close the treatment gap, in some cases.

In addition to competing needs such as child care and transportation, health plan interviewees identified homelessness and co-occurring mental disorders as factors that compete with attention to SUD treatment. Those who are homeless can be difficult to reach, and being homeless makes treatment attendance more difficult. Although health plans do not pay for housing, care managers and outreach workers can and do work with beneficiaries to assist in obtaining housing that can facilitate treatment. Similarly, co-occurring mental illness can impede treatment initiation and engagement [156], because mental illness and SUD negatively affect each other if both are not addressed. Yet, a person's ability to attend to both may be limited. Health plan efforts to identify and implement initiatives that integrate SUD and mental health care services seek to provide improved ease of access for care that addresses co-occurring conditions. These and other potentially competing needs get in the way of treatment participation. Increased focus on social determinants of health by health plans requires resources that many may not have.

As the literature indicates [12], stigma is a powerful barrier to care, and plans that have reached out to educate communities about SUD and the positive effects of treatment are taking steps to alleviate stigma. Nearly all of the plan representatives with whom we met mentioned the issue of stigma associated with SUD. Individuals may feel stigmatized by attitudes in the community, by providers, or even by their own family, which may prevent them from seeking treatment or, sometimes, even acknowledging the problem.

Competing Needs

Women historically have been more difficult to engage in SUD treatment. Competing needs such as transportation and child care may play a role. Addressing those issues may facilitate increased initiation and engagement for women.

Plans have reached out to educate communities about SUD and the positive effects of treatment, seeking to alleviate such stigma. This education also may increase patient activation, which is a contributor to treatment participation [62]. Plan representatives also cited instances in which plans can provide SUD treatment that is fully integrated into treatment for physical health as examples of successfully circumventing fears associated with stigma.

Patients who do not have to enter a building specifically designated as an SUD treatment facility but instead can use the same facilities where they access other medical care are less fearful of being identified as in SUD treatment. Co-locating SUD and physical health treatment, however, often is in the hands of providers rather than plans. Integrated systems and small plans that incorporate providers appear better suited to address the physical manifestations of care that may alleviate stigma than do larger plans that contract with a host of providers in various care settings and that may have difficulty filling their networks regardless of care coordination or co-location capacity. It seems, however, that efforts to integrate care, co-locate services, and provide education all can serve to both help alleviate stigma and address conditions that co-occur with SUD.

The literature indicates that younger people in particular may be more comfortable with a harm reduction approach to treatment than with an abstinence-based approach [124]. To address the fact that many patients may not be ready to abstain from substance use, health plans increasingly are shifting their approach to promoting harm reduction environments rather than abstinence-driven programs. The need to engage people in treatment, even if the goal is harm reduction, is important when the only alternative may be continued use at high rates, resulting in overdose and exposure to additional health risks.

Provider Influences on SUD Treatment Participation

Provider characteristics also were identified as influencing treatment initiation and engagement. Many health plan interviewees reported feeling that provider stigma about treating patients with an SUD, or Medicaid patients generally, interfered with providers' ability or desire to encourage members to initiate SUD treatment. Related to this provider stigma is provider discomfort with the subject matter and lack of expertise. Previous research suggests that many PCPs do not feel competent about their ability to treat patients with an SUD. Physicians cite a lack of addictions-focused training, personal stigma, and time constraints as limiting their ability to screen for SUD or link patients with risky behavior to treatment services [13, 14, 15].

Many health plan representatives interviewed in the present study described developing a variety of educational opportunities directed at enhancing providers' knowledge of SUD issues in general, as well as evidence-based and other best practices for substance use screening and treatment. However, one plan expressed reluctance to target initiatives to providers because plan staff members fear overwhelming providers with information on new initiatives, tools, and other SUD-related information. This plan seemed to focus its efforts more extensively on patients than on providers, whereas the remainder of plans attempted both. Upon reviewing the relative rankings of this plan with the others on IET, researchers found initiation in the 85th percentile and engagement in the 95th percentile, with good performance on other behavioral health measures as well. This limited information does not allow any conclusion to be drawn on the preferability of one approach over the other.

Provider shortages also are a factor that can limit SUD treatment initiation and engagement. For example, 53 percent of all counties in the United States lack any waivered buprenorphine prescribers [87]. These and other shortages were mentioned throughout the interviews as impeding access to care. Efforts that plans do make to address provider expertise and attitudes logically should alleviate provider shortages to some extent as well. Plans did describe outreach and other approaches to induce providers into their networks; however, solving the problem of provider shortages clearly is not simple, given absolute provider shortages, providers only accepting cash, and other factors impeding adequate coverage of beneficiary needs. Shortages of individual providers such as addiction specialists, psychiatrists, and buprenorphine prescribers, as well as residential treatment, detox facilities, or OPTs, combine to make access to the right level of care at the right time difficult for many plan beneficiaries. To some extent, these shortages are associated with the lack of available expertise and provider desire to work with patients with an SUD. They also pertain to network adequacy – a factor discussed later regarding health plan-related factors influencing initiation and engagement. However, addressing workforce shortages and adequacy of reimbursement and working to reduce stigma are important to alleviate shortages. Further, finding incentives to encourage providers to accept insurance or to deincentivize the demand for cash is worth exploring to boost the inventory of available providers for individuals with an SUD.

Market and Environmental Influences on SUD Treatment Participation

Existing literature indicates that SUD treatment gaps often are found in the South, Southwest, or Midwest and that OUD treatment gaps are greatest in the Great Plains and in the Southeast [87]. As a result, the current study aimed to interview health plans in geographically diverse locations including the Northeast, Southeast, Midwest, and West. Geographic and policy elements interact within this study because two of the interviewed Medicaid plans operate under state policies that have not expanded Medicaid eligibility and benefits in response to the Affordable Care Act – with one located in the Southeast and the other in the Northern Midwest region. Although both of these non-expansion Medicaid plans were higher performers on the IET measures, more limited Medicaid coverage may have positively affected initiation and engagement rates by eliminating substantial segments of the population with an SUD who might have been covered in other states. Further, because of limitations in the state Medicaid plan, one of the plans in a non-expansion state did not reimburse for certain services (e.g., IOP and partial hospitalization, peer services) that were routinely covered services for plans located in expansion states.

In the qualitative component of this study, health plan interviewees identified two national policies as significantly influencing treatment participation. Many interviewees cited the regulation at 42 CFR Part 2 as interfering with plans' abilities to coordinate care, most often with detox facilities or specialty substance use inpatient facilities. One plan representative hypothesized that specialty facilities are more familiar with the regulation and thus more hesitant to share information about admission or treatment for SUDs, whereas general hospitals may be less aware of 42 CFR Part 2 and more likely to operate under the assumption that the standard confidentiality provisions apply to all services.

Interviewees from two different health plans made it clear that they regarded the recent amendment to the regulation as having "wasted an opportunity" to expand the ability of health plans to coordinate care for their enrollees. To address this issue, some plans impose prior authorization or notification requirements that allow them to know in advance that an enrollee will be admitted, permitting them to follow up. Others are involved in extensive efforts to work closely with detox facilities or hospitals to ensure that there is an ongoing close relationship and trust and to facilitate systems that permit notification of enrollee admission that will allow timely follow-up. In an era when efforts are being made to get away from prior authorization in the treatment of SUD, it appears that it does have a role to play in situations such as this, although notification rather than authorization may be a subtle difference with fewer reimbursement repercussions. Rather than being required to engage in these workarounds, however, health plans clearly would prefer either that the regulation be amended or that the provider community better understand that plans' ability to know what is happening with their beneficiaries is critical to effective care coordination. The plans obviously see themselves as responsible for care coordination and perceive the regulation as a substantial barrier impeding their ability to carry out that responsibility.

Another federal policy mentioned was the restriction on Medicaid coverage of care in IMDs. Only one of the five representatives from Medicaid plans we interviewed discussed trying to identify residential facilities with fewer than 16 beds in order to provide their members access to Medicaid-reimbursable residential treatment. Representatives from this Medicaid plan and the one commercial plan interviewed both expressed frustration over the limited number of residential treatment beds available in their communities, regardless of IMD constraints. Under the current Section 1115 SUD delivery system waivers, an increasing number of Medicaid plans will be able to reimburse for residential treatment [20]. However, access may remain limited because of a general shortage of residential treatment capacity. Given that bivariate results from the quantitative analyses indicated that the commercial plans reimbursing for residential treatment had higher rates of treatment initiation, one hopes that the loosening of reimbursement might encourage an increase in the number of beds available if payment is an option.

Analyses revealed different ways in which state policies and other state characteristics influence treatment initiation and engagement. For example, multivariate analyses indicated that higher rates of initiation of OUD treatment were associated with being in a state with a higher-than-average prevalence of opioid prescriptions in relation to the state's population. This finding is logical, assuming that higher rates of opioid prescribing are associated with higher rates of OUD and higher demand for OUD treatment.

In quantitative analyses, initiation of OUD treatment also was negatively associated with being in a state where prescribers or dispensers are required to access the PDMP in certain circumstances. This result simply may mean that identifying problems with opioid prescribing or identifying doctor or pharmacy shopping does not translate to referral to OUD treatment. Interviews with health plan representatives revealed mixed perspectives on the utility of PDMPs. Interviewees reported significant variation in PDMP use in states without laws requiring PDMP consultation prior to prescribing, dispensing, or both. However, plans generally expressed a desire to use data in ways that would allow them to better identify problems of misuse and target treatment initiation and engagement efforts toward those identified as obtaining inappropriate controlled substance prescriptions. Although health plans can and do use their own claims data for information on prescription fills paid by the plan, access to PDMP data would allow the plans to know whether beneficiaries were filling excessive or unnecessary prescriptions and paying for them with cash, thereby circumventing plan lock-in policies. Recent research using PDMP data has revealed that the implementation of pharmacy lock-ins may result in increased out-of-pocket payment for prescription opioids [157], supporting plan arguments that access to those data would be useful in curtailing opioid misuse.

Interviews with health plans revealed additional circumstances in which state policies may impede or facilitate SUD initiation or engagement. For example, state Medicaid agencies limit what their associated Medicaid health plans can reimburse for services such as peer support and recovery services. Some plans accept this state benefit restriction, whereas others find ways to help beneficiaries access peer services in the community. State Medicaid policies that allow beneficiaries to frequently switch plans also were identified as impeding plans' abilities to coordinate services and as permitting patient evasion of plans' pharmacy lock-in policies. One state was reported to have imposed additional limitations on the freedom of Medicaid beneficiaries to change plans, thereby mitigating some "plan-shopping." Low Medicaid reimbursement rates and, in one case, substantially delayed reimbursement from the state agency, also were identified as significant factors limiting plans' ability to expand network adequacy and ensure access to care for beneficiaries. Medicaid plans expressed concern that providers withhold open spots from Medicaid beneficiaries so they can receive greater reimbursement rates from commercial plan members and individuals paying out-of-pocket. States struggle with these factors that stem from state Medicaid policies and, ultimately, budgetary considerations that impede the ability of Medicaid plans to engage providers and serve their beneficiaries.

State policies that provide for coverage of MAT or that preclude the use of prior authorization for MAT or other SUD services can encourage easier access to needed treatments and facilitate initiation and engagement in treatment. As noted earlier, however, plan use of prior authorizations for notification purposes can facilitate treatment if it has the effect of alerting the plan to patient admission to a detox facility in real time, thereby allowing follow-up prior to discharge and subsequent initiation or engagement in step-down treatment. Unfortunately, use of prior authorization also may have the effect of making prescribing sufficiently more difficult if it creates an unnecessary barrier to care.

Health Plan Influences on SUD Treatment Participation

Our review of the literature found three overarching types of health plan interventions that have been used to improve initiation and engagement in SUD treatment: (1) implementation of evidence-based clinical practices; (2) interventions that may better address the needs of special populations; and (3) organizational interventions. Our quantitative analyses and analysis of health plan interviews provided us with additional insight into these three categories. As already mentioned, health plans may focus some of their quality improvement efforts on increasing provider knowledge of SUDs and SUD treatment and on accelerating use of evidence-based practices, including MAT. Health plan interventions that address the needs of special populations may include interventions: (1) in collaboration with schools or with local law enforcement or other correctional systems; or (2) that focus on women who are pregnant or parenting or on beneficiaries who are homeless. Health plans also must take account of variable substance use in their populations. For example, identifying beneficiaries at moderate risk of having an SUD may be difficult, and plans increasingly are using pharmaceutical claims mining to find individuals, for instance, who are obtaining excessive opioid prescriptions and targeting outreach to those individuals, as well as imposing pharmacy or provider lock-ins. This drug utilization review approach is supported by CMS [20] and is advocated as part of the HFPP. The HFPP encourages the use of data, among other things, to identify patients at risk of opioid misuse and OUD and to intervene on the basis of those findings [142]. Further, although opioid use receives the most attention, alcohol remains the drug used most pervasively and, in some areas, other drugs such as cocaine or methamphetamine are commonly used, and individual health plans must find ways to address related use disorders appropriately.

Both quantitative and qualitative analyses identified organizational-related interventions as significant factors in increasing treatment uptake. Some of the current study's reported findings echo those identified in the existing literature, but we also gathered considerable new information, providing insights into strategies and structures of health plans that are successful at initiating and engaging beneficiaries into SUD treatment.

Interventions

Our review of the literature found 3 overarching types of health plan interventions that have been used to improve initiation and engagement in SUD treatment: (1) implementation of evidence-based clinical practices; (2) interventions that may better address the needs of special populations; and (3) organizational interventions.

Health Plan Structure

Bivariate quantitative analyses showed that plans with the largest numbers of beneficiaries tended to have the lowest rates of initiation and engagement for both SUD and OUD, as did plans with higher percentages of beneficiaries with an SUD or an OUD. To some extent, this result may be explained by observations from the health plan interviews. The health plan representatives we interviewed were from one small local plan, four medium-sized regional plans, and one large national plan. All but the small local plan had a multilevel system of governance, with both corporate and local oversight of mental health care and SUD services and different degrees of local versus enterprise-level oversight of utilization management, care management, care coordination, and quality improvement. However, all the regional or national insurance companies stressed that some level of local decision-making was critical to implementing behavioral health policies and procedures in ways that responded to local population needs. These plans relied heavily on local leadership, with state-specific plan presidents, medical directors, and behavioral health directors overseeing regionally stationed case management and care coordination teams. Interviewees repeatedly endorsed regular communication between corporate and local leadership, as well as internal communication at the local level, as critical to address beneficiary needs or access challenges. A locally focused approach with ample communication may be one of the ways in which the plans selected for interviewing differentiate themselves from others that may fare more poorly on initiation and engagement, if lack of local governance and local initiatives are more limited among the latter.

Although the national plan interviewees indicated that their plan depended more on corporate oversight and noted that their approach enabled them to streamline decision-making and ensure consistency across their business lines, the results of their IET rates were not distinguishable from those of the other plans interviewed. It may be more telling, however, that only one of the six plans interviewed had a clearly more centralized approach, suggesting either that smaller plans are simply more willing to submit to interviews or that a localized approach is more likely to place a plan in the upper echelons of IET results. Without better understanding of the governance of poorly performing plans, conclusions cannot be drawn regarding whether a more locally focused approach is preferable.

Reimbursement and Benefit Design

It appears that the provision of more components of the SUD care continuum influence initiation and engagement rates. Multivariate quantitative analyses showed that higher-performing health plans for both SUD and OUD initiation and engagement provided more IOP or partial hospitalization services than did lower-performing plans. SUD engagement was associated with increased outpatient services as well, whereas, in bivariate analyses, provision of residential services was linked to higher initiation rates. Representatives from the six plans that we interviewed all discussed the importance of reimbursing for the full SUD care continuum. Plan interviewees frequently compared the extent of their SUD service benefit with their ability to bring members into SUD care services. When more intensive services such as partial hospitalization and residential treatment were unavailable, some health plan representatives described finding other creative ways to engage members in inpatient, outpatient and community-based recovery support services. Although the state Medicaid agency sets service benefits for five of the interviewed plans, some of their leadership and care coordination teams viewed benefit design as having some mutability and capacity for augmentation via community partnerships through coordination of a patchwork of available services to substitute for unavailable treatment options.

Quantitative analyses indicated that out-of-pocket costs and provider reimbursement are other factors affecting treatment uptake. Our multivariate analyses found that commercial plans with higher rates of SUD treatment initiation had higher-than-average median out-of-pocket costs for outpatient SUD services per user. Bivariate analyses showed similar associations between higher performance on SUD initiation and engagement and higher out-of-pocket outpatient costs and outpatient reimbursement. The same was largely true for OUD treatment. These results may not necessarily mean that those commercial plans imposed higher co-pays or deductibles. Indeed, bivariate analyses showed that high-deductible plans fared more poorly on the IET rates. Instead, it may mean that, for those who require SUD services, more services are provided and, with each of those services, a co-pay accrues, increasing the overall out-of-pocket cost to the person for multiple aspects of treatment. This interpretation makes sense, given that a higher quantity of outpatient services per beneficiary also was associated with better initiation and engagement. There is, however, no assurance that the same result would be obtained in a Medicaid population, and the high performing Medicaid plans examined in this study did not require any out-of-pocket expenditures. Medicaid plans also generally reported not requiring members to face out-of-pocket costs for services available only from out-of-network providers. When out-of-network providers were identified as necessary, the health plan representatives reported either contracting with the provider to come into network or making special one-time arrangements to reimburse for services at no costs to members.

In contrast to outpatient results, bivariate results showed that inpatient out-of-pocket costs and reimbursement were lower for commercial plans that did better on SUD and OUD initiation and engagement. This suggests that plans that rely more on intensive and more costly inpatient services are not successfully taking that next step of initiating beneficiaries into treatment and finding ways to keep them in treatment. Thus, rather than reimburse for less-costly outpatient services, these lower-performing plans may rely more on hospitalization and little else.

There were paradoxical results among the bivariate analyses related to costs and reimbursement of MAT as part of OUD treatment, all of which potentially provide evidence that improved coverage of MAT is associated with improved initiation and engagement in OUD treatment. Higher rates of OUD treatment initiation were associated with higher out-of-pocket costs and higher pharmacy reimbursement for MAT medications, which may relate either to higher co-pays within the commercial plans or to more permissive induction dosing with accompanying higher costs. In contrast, higher rates of engagement were associated with lower out-of-pocket costs and pharmacy reimbursement for MAT medications, suggesting that, for commercial patients, longer-term use of MAT may be more price sensitive. Bivariate analyses of duration of MAT treatment found that higher-performing plans on both initiation and engagement in OUD treatment more commonly reimbursed longer periods of MAT treatment (more than 14 days) than did lower-performing plans. Among the health plans interviewed, all covered at least two opioid MAT drug options – all covered buprenorphine or buprenorphine-naloxone and methadone. In other words, all of the health plans selected for interview perceive MAT to be an integral part of treatment and treat it accordingly within their reimbursement structure.

Network Adequacy

On the basis of distance and number of providers proximate to beneficiaries, health plans impose internal standards and/or must meet state requirements for network adequacy. Although the health plan representatives interviewed reported satisfying their requirements, all indicated that these requirements are not always sufficient to ensure adequate access. Many of these requirements related to the number of addiction specialists, buprenorphine or methadone prescribers, and detox and residential facilities.

Health plan representatives interviewed consistently stated that finding buprenorphine prescribers for beneficiaries often was difficult. Many areas lacked waivered prescribers and, where there were waivered prescribers, many did not accept patients or did not accept Medicaid patients, often preferring cash payments. Health plan interviewees described efforts to expand their MAT provider networks, and one health plan interviewee reported conducting monthly outreach to assess which buprenorphine prescribers are accepting new patients. Methadone availability also sometimes was lacking. The small Medicaid plan had worked with a methadone provider located elsewhere in the state to open a new OTP in a town near the plan's center of operations, allowing enhanced access for its beneficiaries. Detox facilities and residential treatment facilities for placement after detox also often were lacking. Even though most plans could not reimburse for residential treatment, if payment was available from other sources, treatment settings sometimes were not. When asked about use of telehealth to expand capacity, several plans reported not using it for SUD treatment.

These findings suggest both that alternative approaches to assessing network adequacy and that alternative approaches to ensuring treatment access deserve further attention from researchers and policymakers. If SUD treatment is cost-effective, investing in options for treatment access makes sense to further treatment access and to conserve overall resources.

Integration, Care Coordination, and Care Management

All health plans interviewed have taken significant steps toward integrating care, including physical health, mental health, and SUD treatment. These steps range from conducting patient-focused and provider-focused interventions such as requiring universal mental health and substance use screening by physical health providers or co-locating SUD counseling services in physical health settings to internal plan-focused efforts that involve team meetings that can address multiple aspects of individual beneficiaries' needs. Interviewees clearly took a holistic view of member needs and were focused on collaborative efforts between plan leadership, clinicians, and plan members.

> **Integrated Care**
>
> One of the primary tools to facilitate integrated care, as well as improve initiation and engagement in SUD treatment, was the use of plan-based care coordinators, care managers, and outreach workers.

One of the primary tools used to facilitate integrated care, as well as improved initiation and engagement in SUD treatment, was the use of plan-based care coordinators, care managers, and outreach workers. Interviewed plans placed an emphasis on maintaining a balance of such staff members who relied on phone contact and others who worked with beneficiaries in the community, including conducting house calls or meeting them in hospitals or detox facilities.

Several health plans also promoted cross-system integration by working with schools, law enforcement, providers for homeless individuals, or services for pregnant women.

These health plan care management and coordination positions, and the staff efforts to augment reimbursed services, integrate care, and pull individuals with an SUD into treatment, are clearly critical to allowing the currently high performing plans to do well on the IET measure. Increasing mechanisms to pay for care coordination and management, as well as cross-system integration, will be important to improve SUD treatment initiation and engagement across a broader range of payers beyond these that are currently higher-performing.

Quality Improvement Initiatives

Health plans reported investing significant resources in quality improvement activities, expressing a concern that poorly managed SUDs would result in higher overall costs for the plan and inadequate care for beneficiaries. Quality improvement efforts have included developing new staff positions to support activities, investing in software to develop data analytic capabilities including data mining, and facilitating secure communication with beneficiaries and providers.

Although plans that are not provider owned did not engage in shared savings with providers, two interviewees mentioned plans to begin, possibly as a pilot or as part of a state Medicaid ACO initiative. A number of the plans, however, are themselves subject to alternative payment models such as value-based payment or pay-for-performance models designed to incentivize desired behaviors or outcomes as part of quality improvement. In the case of Medicaid plans, a state will establish certain performance measures (e.g., IET or follow-up after hospitalization) as metrics to which payment may attach. States may implement shared savings, whereby higher performance results in payment to the plan, and/or may tie metrics to payment withholds, whereby the health plan is penalized financially should it fail to meet predetermined state benchmarks on SUD measures.

Two of the Medicaid plans reported focusing their time and financial investments on initiatives that targeted activities related to quality measures for which they were financially at risk under the state Medicaid plan. They are very motivated to maximize their returns on those metrics.

Plans described organizing leadership, contracting teams, and member outreach employees to develop and engage in extensive, measure-focused innovations that target multiple aspects of health plan organization, communication strategies, and relationship building with providers and beneficiaries. Health plans also closely attend to the importance of changing their approach and being sensitive to state-directed modifications to measures and payment arrangements. As states shift their emphasis to new measures or redesign the way in which benchmark metrics can be achieved, plans are actively adjusting their approach and identifying new ways to meet these expectations.

This raises three issues for policymakers:

1) Health plans that are not doing well on initiation and engagement either may not be subject to a pay-for-performance model or may completely lack the resources to respond, and policymakers should understand and address either circumstance.
2) The measures that policymakers select to incentivize must be measures that really assess something that is very important to encourage because the focus on those measures may reduce focus in other important but unincentivized areas.
3) Removal of a good measure from the group to which incentives attach may result in loss of focus and declining performance if the initiatives undertaken to improve performance on that measure no longer are sustained.

Study Limitations

Although this expansive mixed-methods study presents and synthesizes valuable quantitative and qualitative data, like all studies it has limitations. The rapid change that has taken place in recent years in health care generally, and in behavioral health care in particular, means that managed care plans identified for potential interviews based on 2014 results on the IET measure were somewhat different when staff members were interviewed in 2017. Plan personnel, plan structure, and plan initiatives all changed in the intervening 3 years. Thus, the positive rates of initiation and engagement in 2014, as well as plan strategies for improving SUD treatment participation, may have continued, grown, or decreased. This means that information gathered in interviews represents more closely the status in 2017 than that in 2014.

Another limitation related to the mixed-methods approach involves the fact that the quantitative analyses used commercial insurance data, yet the qualitative interviews were primarily with Medicaid plans. Obtaining access to representatives of high performing commercial plans for interviews was much more difficult than scheduling interviews with representatives of Medicaid plans. Although this limitation represents a difference between the quantitative and qualitative aspects of the study, it may provide the benefit of balancing the information gathered.

Finally, some variables used in the quantitative analyses may not have completely captured the sort of information that was intended, particularly among the market and environmental characteristics variables. For example, the variable *Buprenorphine Prescribers*, which relies on the SAMHSA website listing waivered buprenorphine prescribers [149], captures imperfect information about the number of buprenorphine prescribers actually available and taking patients. Evidence from our interviews with health plans clearly indicates that many waivered prescribers do not accept any patients or accept less than their limit, and that many who do accept patients simultaneously do not accept insurance and require payment in cash. The link between high performing health plans and this state-level variable also is attenuated by the fact that high performance on IET does not include MAT (e.g., buprenorphine) as treatment and relies instead on counseling and other non-medication services, which high performing plans in areas with few prescribers may actually rely on more heavily to compensate for the inability of their enrollees to easily access MAT. Similarly, *SSA Spending* – which was intended to indicate level of state support for SUDs but actually captures only a portion of resources available within states – is an imperfect proxy for market or policy realities.

CONCLUSION

Identifying mechanisms to enhance SUD treatment initiation and continued engagement in care is a public health priority. Although more than 20.8 million Americans have a diagnosed need for SUD treatment, few access or complete appropriate treatment [1, 2]. As both administrators and coordinators of health care benefits, health plans are positioned to play a crucial role in mitigating potential access barriers and developing facilitating mechanisms that bring beneficiaries into care and keep them there.

This study sought to identify which health plan characteristics – including models of care, interventions, and best practices – are associated with achieving high rates of initiation and engagement in SUD treatment. We aimed to examine additional market factors – including health policies, provider availability, and population characteristics – that affect performance on these measures. Sequential, mixed-method analyses yielded core understandings of how health plans navigate obstacles and leverage opportunities to bring members into SUD treatment and maintain engagement over time.

The following are some ways in which health plans have the potential to address several key barriers while leveraging additional facilitators to achieve high rates of initiation and engagement in SUD treatment. Many of these reflect initiatives undertaken by the higher-performing plans interviewed; others are options that may address some of the barriers identified but not resolved:

- Coordinating assistance and entitlements for members with competing social demands including childcare, transportation, and housing that otherwise prevent them from attending treatment appointments.
- Integrating service provision and coordinating treatment plans to address members' holistic physical and behavioral health needs in ways that respond to member-identified priorities.
- Augmenting provider and outreach staff knowledge of the SUD care continuum and recovery process.

- Implementing care models that support routine check-ins with members about their readiness for behavior change and include a spectrum of services from harm reduction to more intensive treatment levels that can bring more members into care over time.
- Developing provider-focused and community-focused campaigns to combat stigma around SUDs and to promote treatment-seeking behaviors, with greater support for members contemplating treatment and for those engaging in the recovery process.
- Cultivating health plan outreach staff knowledge of and relationships with community-based recovery support services to provide members with additional services beyond the benefit array.
- Engaging with treatment facilities in educational opportunities that alleviate misinterpretations of federal privacy regulations such as 42 CFR Part 2 to encourage a common legal understanding of information-sharing restrictions that do not unnecessarily hinder health plan outreach and care coordination efforts.
- Investing resources in developing capabilities for data analytics and responsive activities that accurately respond to the measured needs of members.
- Scheduling routine communication opportunities between health plan leadership, quality improvement teams, contracting teams, and SUD-focused and mental health-focused teams, including outreach workers and case managers.

Ongoing in-depth examinations of barriers and facilitators to treatment uptake are necessary to continue to understand effective methods of enhancing access to recovery services and supports for the thousands of individuals in need of care. SUD trends change over time. This analysis placed a substantial focus on understanding the specific influences that affect treatment uptake for individuals with an OUD because of the current opioid epidemic.

Future research is needed to continue assessing core variables that affect initiation and engagement as drug use patterns evolve and new evidence-based practices are implemented. Close monitoring of how health plan and market characteristics affect access and the efficacy of treatment are crucial to developing processes and models of care that promote and sustain long-term recovery.

REFERENCES

[1] Substance Abuse and Mental Health Services Administration (SAMHSA), Center for Behavioral Health Statistics and Quality. *Key Substance Use and Mental Health Indicators in the United States: Results from the 2015 National Survey on Drug Use and Health.* Publication No. SMA 16-4984, NSDUH Series H-51. Rockville, MD: SAMHSA; 2016.

[2] Substance Abuse and Mental Health Services Administration (SAMHSA), Center for Behavioral Health Statistics and Quality. *2015 National Survey on Drug Use and Health: Detailed Tables Prevalence Estimates, Standard Errors, P Values, and Sample Sizes.* Rockville, MD: SAMHSA; 2016.

[3] Centers for Disease Control and Prevention (CDC*). Prescription Opioid Overdose Data. CDC website.* Atlanta, GA: CDC. Updated August 1, 2017. https://www.cdc.gov/drugoverdose/data/overdose.html. Accessed September 21, 2017.

[4] Substance Abuse and Mental Health Services Administration (SAMHSA), Center for Behavioral Health Statistics and Quality. *Behavioral Health Trends in the United States: Results from the 2014 National Survey on Drug Use and Health.* Publication No. SMA 15-4927, NSDUH Series H-50. Rockville, MD: SAMHSA; 2015.

[5] Substance Abuse and Mental Health Services Administration (SAMHSA), Office of Applied Studies. Treatment Episode Data Set (TEDS), *2006: Discharges from Substance Abuse Treatment Services.* DASIS Series: S-46, HHS Publication No. (SMA) 09-4378. Rockville, MD: SAMHSA; 2009.

[6] *Analysis of Medicaid HEDIS data by the National Committee for Quality Assurance, as presented in the CMS Medicaid Innovation Accelerator Program Substance Use Disorder (SUD) Targeted Learning Opportunities Webinar 15 on State of SUD-Related Quality Metrics.* July 11, 2016. https://www.medicaid.gov/state-resource-center/innovation-accelerator-program/iap-downloads/07112016-iap-sud-tlo15.pdf. Accessed September 21, 2017.

[7] Acevedo A, Garnick DW, Lee MT, et al. Racial and ethnic differences in substance abuse treatment initiation and engagement. *J Ethn Subst Abuse*. 2012; 11(1): 1-21. doi:10.1080/15332640.2012.652516.

[8] Fingerhood MI, King VL, Brooner RK, Rastegar DA. A comparison of characteristics and outcomes of opioid-dependent patients initiating office-based buprenorphine or methadone maintenance treatment. *Subst Abus*. 2014; 35(2): 22-126. doi:10.1080/08897077.2013.819828.

[9] Ilgen MA, Price AM, Burnett-Zeigler I, et al. Longitudinal predictors of addictions treatment utilization in treatment-naïve adults with alcohol use disorders. *Drug Alcohol Depend.* 2011; 113(2-3): 215-221. doi:10.1016/j.drugalcdep.2010.08.006.

[10] Resko SM, Mendoza NS. Early attrition from treatment among women with co-occurring substance use disorders and PTSD. *J Soc Work Pract Addict*. 2012; 12(4): 348-369. doi:10.1080/1533256X.2012.728104.

[11] Brown CH, Bennett ME, Li L, Bellack AS. Predictors of initiation and engagement in substance abuse treatment among individuals with co-occurring serious mental illness and substance use disorders. *Addict Behav*. 2011; 36(5): 439-447. doi:10.1016/j.addbeh.2010.12.001.

[12] U.S. Department of Health and Human Services (HHS), Office of the Surgeon General. *Facing Addiction in America: The Surgeon General's Report on Alcohol, Drugs, and Health.* HHS Publication No. (SMA) 16-4991. Washington, DC: Office of the Surgeon General; 2016.

[13] Miller NS, Sheppard LM, Colenda CC, Magen J. Why physicians are unprepared to treat patients who have alcohol-and drug-related disorders. *Acad Med*. 2001; 76(5): 410-418. doi:10.1097/00001888-200105000-00007.

[14] Saitz R, Sullivan L, Samet J. Training community-based clinicians in screening and brief intervention for substance abuse problems: Translating evidence into practice. *Subst Abus*. 2000; 21(1): 21-31. doi:10.1023/A:1007755817351.

[15] Polydorou S, Gunderson EW, Levin FR. Training physicians to treat substance use disorders. *Curr Psychiatry Rep*. 2008; 10(5): 399-404. doi:10.1007/s11920-008-0064-8.

[16] van Boekel LC, Brouwers EPM, van Weeghel J, Garretsen HFL. Stigma among health professionals towards patients with substance use disorders and its consequences for healthcare delivery: Systematic review. *Drug Alcohol Depend*. 2013; 131(1-2): 23-35. doi:10.1016/j.drugalcdep.2013.02.018.

[17] Knudsen HK, Roman PM, Oser CB. Facilitating factors and barriers to the use of medications in publicly funded addiction treatment organizations. *J Addict Med*. 2010; 4(2): 99-107. doi:10.1097/ADM.0b013e3181b41a32.

[18] Arfken CL, Johanson C-E, di Menza S, Schuster CR. Expanding treatment capacity for opioid dependence with office-based treatment with buprenorphine: National surveys of physicians. *J Subst Abuse Treat*. 2010; 39(2): 96-104. doi:10.1016/j.jsat.2010.05.004.

[19] Dick AW, Pacula RL, Gordon AJ, et al. Growth in buprenorphine waivers for physicians increased potential access to opioid agonist treatment, 2002-11. *Health Aff* (Millwood). 2015; 34(6): 1028-1034. doi:10.1377/hlthaff.2014.1205.

[20] Centers for Medicare & Medicaid Services (CMS). *Medicaid Drug Utilization Review.* State Comparison/Summary Report FFY 2015. Annual Report. Baltimore, MD: CMS; 2016. https://www.medicaid.gov/medicaid-chip-program-information/by-topics/prescription-drugs/downloads/2015-dur-summary-report.pdf. Accessed September 21, 2017.

[21] Weber EW. Failure of physicians to prescribe pharmacotherapies for addiction: Regulatory restrictions and physician resistance. *J Heal Care L Pol'y*. 2010; 13(1): 49-76.

[22] National Center on Addiction and Substance Abuse (CASA). *Uncovering Coverage Gaps: A Review of Addiction Benefits in ACA Plans*. New York, NY: CASA; 2016.

[23] Quinn A, Reif S, Merrick EL, Horgan CM, Garnick DW, Stewart MT. How do private health plans manage specialty behavioral health treatment entry and continuing care? *Psychiatr Serv*. 2017 May 15. [Epub ahead of print]. doi: 10.1176/appi.ps.201600081.

[24] Grogan CM, Andrews C, Abraham A, Humphreys K, Pollack HA, Smith BT, Friedmann PD. Survey highlights differences In Medicaid coverage for substance use treatment and opioid use disorder medications. *Health Aff* (Millwood). 2016;35(12):2289-2296. doi: 10.1377/hlthaff.2016.0623.

[25] Substance Abuse and Mental Health Services Administration (SAMHSA). *Medicaid Coverage and Financing of Medications to Treat Alcohol and Opioid Use Disorders*. HHS Publication No. SMA-14-4854. Rockville, MD: SAMHSA; 2014.

[26] Kelly TM, Daley DC. Integrated treatment of substance use and psychiatric disorders. *Soc Work Public Health*. 2013; 28(3-4): 388-406. doi:10.1080/19371918.2013.774673.

[27] Schaefer JA, Cronkite RC, Hu KU. Differential relationships between continuity of care practices, engagement in continuing care, and abstinence among subgroups of patients with substance use and psychiatric disorders. *J Stud Alcohol Drugs*. 2011; 72(4): 611-621. doi:10.15288/jsad.2011.72.611.

[28] McLellan AT, Chalk M, Bartlett J. Outcomes, performance, and quality: What's the difference? *J Subst Abuse Treat*. 2007; 32(4): 331-340. doi:10.1016/j.jsat.2006.09.004.

[29] National Committee for Quality Assurance (NCQA). *The State of Health Care Quality 2013: Improving Quality and Patient Experience*. 2013. Washington, DC: NCQA; 2013. https://www.ncqa.org/Portals/0/Newsroom/SOHC/2013/SOHC-web_version_report.pdf. Accessed September 21, 2017.

[30] Han B, Gfroerer JC, Colliver JD, Penne MA. Substance use disorder among older adults in the United States in 2020. *Addiction*. 2009; 104(1): 88-96. doi:10.1111/j.1360-0443.2008.02411.x.

[31] Grant BF, Goldstein RB, Saha TD, et al. Epidemiology of DSM-5 alcohol use disorder: Results from the National Epidemiologic Survey on Alcohol and Related Conditions III. *JAMA Psychiatry*. 2015; 72(8): 757-766. doi:10.1001/jamapsychiatry.2015.0584.

[32] FAIR Health. *The Impact of the Opioid Crisis on the Healthcare System: A Study of Privately Billed Services*. New York, NY: FAIR Health; 2016.

[33] Substance Abuse and Mental Health Services Administration (SAMHSA). *Center for Behavioral Health Statistics and Quality. Results from the 2013 National Survey on Drug Use and Health:* Detailed Tables. Rockville, MD: SAMHSA; 2013.

[34] Jones CM, Logan J, Gladden R, Bohm MK. Vital Signs: Demographic and substance use trends among heroin users – United States, 2002-2013. *Morb Mortal Wkly Rep*. 2015; 64(26): 719-725.

[35] Gryczynski J, Schwartz RP, O'Grady KE, Restivo L, Mitchell SG, Jaffe JH. Understanding patterns of high-cost health care use across different substance user groups. *Health Aff* (Millwood). 2016; 35(1): 12-19. doi:10.1377/hlthaff.2015.0618.

[36] Centers for Disease Control and Prevention (CDC). *Heroin Overdose Data.* CDC website. Atlanta, GA: CDC. Updated January 26, 2017. https://www.cdc.gov/drugoverdose/data/heroin.html. Accessed September 21, 2017.

[37] Centers for Disease Control and Prevention (CDC). Increases in Heroin Overdose Deaths – 28 States, 2010 to 2012. *Morb Mortalitiy Wkly Rep*. 2014; 63(39): 849-854.

[38] Rudd R, Seth P, David F, Scholl L. Increases in drug and opioid-involved overdose deaths – United States, 2010-2015. *MMWR Morb Mortal Wkly Rep*. 2016; 65(50-51): 1445-1452.

[39] Bondurant SR, Lindo JM, Swenson ID. National Bureau of Economic Research (NBER) Working Paper No. 22610. *Substance Abuse Treatment Centers and Local Crime*. Cambridge, MA: NBER; 2016.

[40] Wen H, Hockenberry JM, Cummings JR. National Bureau of Economic Research (NBER) Working Paper No. 20537. *The Effect of Substance Use Disorder Treatment Use on Crime: Evidence from Public Insurance Expansions and Health Insurance Parity Mandates*. Cambridge, MA: NBER; 2014.

[41] Centers for Disease Control and Prevention (CDC). Alcohol and Public Health: Alcohol-Related Disease Impact (ARDI). *Average for United States 2006-2010 Alcohol-Attributable Deaths Due to Excessive Alcohol Use*. CDC website. Atlanta, GA: CDC; 2013. https://nccd.cdc.gov/DPH_ARDI/Default/Report.aspx?T=AAM&P=f6d7eda7-036e-4553- 9968-9b17ffad620e&R=d7a9b303-48e9-4440-bf47-070a4827e1fd&M=8E1C5233-5640- 4EE8-9247-1ECA7DA325B9&F=&D=. Accessed September 21, 2017.

[42] Bouchery EE, Harwood HJ, Sacks JJ, Simon CJ, Brewer RD. Economic costs of excessive alcohol consumption in the US, 2006. *Am J Prev Med*. 2011; 41(5): 516–524.

[43] Heilig M, Goldman D, Berrettini W, O'Brien CP. Pharmacogenetic approaches to the treatment of alcohol addiction. *Nat Rev Neurosci*. 2011; 12(11): 670-684. doi:10.1038/nrn3110.

[44] McKay JR, Krandler HR, Kampman KM, Ashare RL, Schnoll RA. Psychopharmacological treatments for substance use disorders. In: Nathan N, JM G, eds. *A Guide to Treatments That Work*. 3rd ed. New York, NY: Oxford University Press; 2015: 763-800.

[45] Lopez-Quintero C, Roth KB, Eaton WW, et al. Mortality among heroin users and users of other internationally regulated drugs: A 27-year follow-up of users in the Epidemiologic Catchment Area Program household samples. *Drug Alcohol Depend*. 2016; 156: 104-111. doi:10.1016/j.drugalcdep.2015.08.030.

[46] PEW Charitable Trusts. *The Case for Medication-Assisted Treatment*. Washington, DC: The Pew Charitable Trusts; 2017. http://www.pewtrusts.org/~/media/assets/2017/02/thecasemedication assistedtreatme nt.pdf. Accessed September 21, 2017.

[47] Florence CS, Zhou C, Luo F, Xu L. The economic burden of prescription opioid overdose, abuse, and dependence in the United States, 2013. *Med Care*. 2016; 54(10): 901-906. doi:10.1097/ MLR.0000000000000625.

[48] Potter JS, Dreifuss JA, Marino EN, et al. The multi-site prescription opioid addiction treatment study: 18-month outcomes. *J Subst Abuse Treat*. 2015; 48(1): 62-69. doi:10.1016/j.jsat.2014.07.009.

[49] Potter JS, Marino EN, Hillhouse MP, et al. Buprenorphine/naloxone and methadone maintenance treatment outcomes for opioid analgesic, heroin, and combined users: Findings from starting treatment with agonist replacement therapies (START). *J Stud Alcohol Drugs*. 2013; 74(4): 605-613.

[50] Nielsen S, Hillhouse M, Thomas C, Hasson A, Ling W. A comparison of buprenorphine taper outcomes between prescription opioid and heroin users. *J Addict Med*. 2013; 7(1): 33-38. doi:10.1097/ADM.0b013e318277e92e.

[51] Hasin DS, Grant BF. The National Epidemiologic Survey on Alcohol and Related Conditions (NESARC) Waves 1 and 2: review and summary of findings. *Soc Psychiatry Psychiatr Epidemiol*. 2015; 50(11): 1609-1640. doi:10.1007/s00127-015-1088-0.

[52] Dreifuss JA, Griffin ML, Frost K, et al. Patient characteristics associated with buprenorphine/naloxone treatment outcome for prescription opioid dependence: Results from a multisite study. *Drug Alcohol Depend*. 2013; 131(1-2): 112-118. doi:10.1016/ j.drugalcdep.2012.12.010.

[53] Mancino M, Curran G, Han X, Allee E, Humphreys K, Booth BM. Predictors of attrition from a national sample of methadone maintenance patients. *Am J Drug Alcohol Abuse*. 2010; 36(3): 155-160. doi:10.3109/00952991003736389.

[54] Gryczynski J, Schwartz RP, Salkever DS, Mitchell SG, Jaffe JH. Patterns in admission delays to outpatient methadone treatment in the United States. *J Subst Abuse Treat*. 2011; 41(4): 431-439. doi:10.1016/j.jsat.2011.06.005.

[55] Saloner B, Lê Cook B. Blacks and Hispanics are less likely than whites to complete addiction treatment, largely due to socioeconomic factors. *Health Aff* (Millwood). 2013; 32(1): 135-145. doi:10.1377/hlthaff.2011.0983.

[56] Lê Cook B, Alegría M. Racial-ethnic disparities in substance abuse treatment: The role of criminal history and socioeconomic status. *Psychiatr Serv*. 2011; 62(11): 1273-1281. doi:10.1176/ps.62.11.pss 6211_1273.

[57] Parran TV, Adelman CA, Merkin B, et al. Long-term outcomes of office-based buprenorphine/naloxone maintenance therapy. *Drug Alcohol Depend*. 2010; 106(1): 56-60. doi:10.1016/j.drugalcdep. 2009.07.013.

[58] Griffin ML, Dodd DR, Potter JS, et al. Baseline characteristics and treatment outcomes in prescription opioid dependent patients with and without co-occurring psychiatric disorder. *Am J Drug Acohol Abus*. 2013; 40(2): 157-162. doi:10.3109/00952990.2013.842241.

[59] Copersino ML, Schretlen DJ, Fitzmaurice G, et al. Effects of cognitive impairment on substance abuse treatment attendance: Predictive validation of a brief cognitive screening measure. *Am J Drug Alcohol Abuse*. 2012; 38(3): 246-250. doi:10.3109/ 00952990.2012.670866.

[60] Hibbard JH, Greene J. What the evidence shows about patient activation: Better health outcomes and care experiences; fewer data on costs. *Health Aff* (Millwood). 2013; 32(2): 207-214. doi:10.1377/hlthaff.2012.1061.

[61] James J. Health Policy Brief: Patient engagement. *Health Aff.* 2013; 36(1). http://www.healthaffairs.org/healthpolicybriefs/brief.php?brief_id=86. Accessed September 21, 2017.

[62] Greene J, Hibbard JH. Why does patient activation matter? An examination of the relationships between patient activation and health-related outcomes. *J Gen Intern Med.* 2012; 27(5): 520-526. doi:10.1007/s11606-011-1931-2.

[63] Shortell SM, Sehgal NJ, Bibi S, et al. An early assessment of accountable care organizations' efforts to engage patients and their families. *Med Care Res Rev.* 2015; 72(5): 580-604. doi:10.1177/1077558715588874.

[64] Mark TL, Lubran R, McCance-Katz EF, Chalk M, Richardson J. Medicaid coverage of medications to treat alcohol and opioid dependence. *J Subst Abuse Treat.* 2015; 55: 1-5. doi:10.1016/j.jsat.2015.04.009.

[65] Substance Abuse and Mental Health Services Administration (SAMHSA). 42 CFR §§ 8.1 *et seq*. Medication Assisted Treatment for Opioid Use Disorders.

[66] Lee MT, Garnick DW, O'Brien PL, et al. Adolescent treatment initiation and engagement in an evidence-based practice initiative. *J Subst Abuse Treat.* 2012; 42(4): 346-355. doi:10.1016/j.jsat.2011.09.005.

[67] Hoffman KA, Ford JH, Tillotson CJ, Choi D, McCarty D. Days to treatment and early retention among patients in treatment for alcohol and drug disorders. *Addict Behav.* 2011; 36(6): 643-647. doi:10.1016/j.addbeh.2011.01.031.

[68] Substance Abuse and Mental Health Services Administration (SAMHSA), *Center for Behavioral Health Statistics and Quality. Treatment Episode Data Set (TEDS): 2002-2012.* National Admissions to Substance Abuse Treatment Services, BHSIS Series S-71, HHS Publication No. (SMA) 14-4850. Rockville, MD: SAMHSA; 2014.

[69] Carroll KM. Dissemination of evidence-based practices: How far we've come, and how much further we've got to go. *Addiction.* 2012; 107(6): 1031-1033. doi:10.1111/j.1360-0443.2011.03755.x.

[70] Fullerton CA, Kim M, Thomas CP, et al. Medication-assisted treatment with methadone: Assessing the evidence. *Psychiatr Serv.* 2014; 65(2): 146-157. doi:10.1176/appi.ps.201300235.

[71] Thomas CP, Fullerton CA, Kim M, et al. Medication-assisted treatment with buprenorphine: Assessing the evidence. *Psychiatr Serv.* 2014; 65(2): 158-170. doi:10.1176/appi.ps.201300256.

[72] McHugh RK, Hearon BA, Otto MW. Cognitive behavioral therapy for substance use disorders. *Psychiatr Clin North Am.* 2010; 33(3). doi:10.1016/j.psc.2010.04.012.

[73] Milward J, Lynskey M, Strang J. Solving the problem of non-attendance in substance abuse services. *Drug Alcohol Rev.* 2014; 33(6): 625-636. doi:10.1111/dar.12194.

[74] Petry NM, Weinstock J, Alessi SM. A randomized trial of contingency management delivered in the context of group counseling. *J Consult Clin Psychol.* 2011; 79(5): 686-696. doi:10.1037/a0024813.

[75] Kidorf M, Brooner RK, Gandotra N, et al. Reinforcing integrated psychiatric service attendance in an opioid-agonist program: A randomized and controlled trial. *Drug Alcohol Depend.* 2013; 133(1): 30-36. doi:10.1016/j.drugalcdep.2013.06.005.

[76] Elwyn G, Dehlendorf C, Epstein RM, Marrin K, White J, Frosch DL. Shared decision making and motivational interviewing: Achieving patient-centered care across the spectrum of health care problems. *Ann Fam Med.* 2014; 12(3): 270-275. doi:10.1370/afm.1615.

[77] Rollnick S, Butler CC, Kinnersley P, Gregory J, Mash B. Motivational interviewing. *BMJ.* 2010; 340(513): c1900. doi:10.1136/bmj.c1900.

[78] Morgenstern J, Kuerbis A, Amrhein P, Hail L, Lynch K, McKay JR. Motivational interviewing: A pilot test of active ingredients and mechanisms of change. *Psychol Addict Behav*. 2012; 26(4): 859-869. doi:10.1037/a0029674.

[79] Kidorf M, King VL, Gandotra N, Kolodner K, Brooner RK. Improving treatment enrollment and re-enrollment rates of syringe exchangers: 12-month outcomes. *Drug Alcohol Depend.* 2012; 124(1-2): 162-166. doi:10.1016/j.drugalcdep.2011.12.008.

[80] Garner BR, Godley SH, Dennis ML, Hunter BD, Bair CML, Godley MD. Using pay for performance to improve treatment implementation for adolescent substance use disorders: Results from a cluster randomized trial. *Arch Pediatr Adolesc Med.* 2012; 166(10): 938-944. doi:10.1001/archpediatrics.2012.802.

[81] Haley SJ, Dugosh KL, Lynch KG. Performance contracting to engage detoxification-only patients into continued rehabilitation. *J Subst Abuse Treat.* 2017; 40(2): 123-131. doi:10.1016 /j.jsat.2010.09.001.

[82] McLellan AT, Kemp J, Brooks A, Carise D. Improving public addiction treatment through performance contracting: The Delaware experiment. *Health Policy*. 2017; 87(3): 296-308. doi:10.1016/ j.healthpol.2008.01.010.

[83] Stewart MT, Horgan CM, Garnick DW, Ritter G, McLellan AT. Performance contracting and quality improvement in outpatient treatment: Effects on waiting time and length of stay. *J Subst Abuse Treat*. 2017; 44(1): 27-33. doi:10.1016/j.jsat.2012.02.001.

[84] Fullerton CA, Henke RM, Crable EL, Hohlbauch A, Cummings N. The impact of medicare acos on improving integration and coordination of physical and behavioral health care. *Health Aff* (Millwood). 2016; 35(7): 1257-1265. doi:10.1377/hlthaff. 2016.0019.

[85] Huskamp H, Barry C. Substance use disorder treatment under new payment and delivery system models. *Paper presented June 24, 2014, at the 5th Biennial Conference of the American Society of Health Economists.* http://ashecon2014.usc.edu/files/2013/07/ASHECON_final.pdf. Accessed September 21, 2017.

[86] Hibbard JH, Greene J, Sacks R, Overton V. Does compensating primary care providers to produce higher quality make them more or less patient centric? *Med Care Res Rev*. 2015; 72(4): 481-495. doi:10.1177/1077558715586291.

[87] Abraham AJ, Andrews CM, Yingling ME, Shannon J. Geographic disparities in availability of opioid use disorder treatment for Medicaid enrollees. *Health Serv Res*. 2017 Mar 27. [Epub ahead of print]. doi: 10.1111/1475-6773.12686.

[88] Cummings JR, Wen H, Ko M. Decline in public substance use disorder treatment centers most serious in counties with high shares of black residents. *Health Aff* (Millwood). 2016; 35(6): 1036-1044. doi:10.1377/hlthaff.2015.1630.

[89] Rosenblatt RA, Andrilla CHA, Catlin M, Larson EH. Geographic and specialty distribution of US physicians trained to treat opioid use disorder. *Ann Fam Med*. 2015; 13(1): 23-26. doi:10.1370/afm.1735.

[90] Levit KR, Mark TL, Coffey RM, et al. Federal spending on behavioral health accelerated during recession as individuals lost employer insurance. *Health Aff* (Millwood). 2013; 32(5): 952-962. doi:10.1377/hlthaff.2012.1065.

[91] Levit KR, Stranges E, Coffey RM, et al. Current and future funding sources for specialty mental health and substance abuse treatment providers. *Psychiatr Serv*. 2013; 64(6): 512-519. doi:10.1176/appi.ps.201200298.

[92] Burns RM, Pacula RL, Bauhoff S, et al. Policies related to opioid agonist therapy for opioid use disorders: The evolution of state policies from 2004 to 2013. *Subst Abus*. 2015; 37(1): 63-69. doi:10.1080/08897077.2015.1080208.

[93] Capoccia VA, Grazier KL, Toal C, Ford JH, Gustafson DH. Massachusetts's experience suggests coverage alone is insufficient to increase addiction disorders treatment. *Health Aff* (Millwood). 2012; 31(5): 1000-1008. doi:10.1377/hlthaff.2011.0326.

[94] Tai B, Volkow ND. Treatment for substance use disorder: Opportunities and challenges under the affordable care act. *Soc Work Public Health*. 2013; 28(3-4): 165-174. doi:10.1080/19371918.2013.758975.

[95] Cummings JR, Wen H, Ko M, Druss BG. Race/Ethnicity and geographic access to Medicaid substance use disorder treatment facilities in the United States. *JAMA Psychiatry*. 2014; 71(2): 190-196. doi:10.1001/jamapsychiatry.2013.3575.

[96] Saloner B, Lê Cook B. An ACA provision increased treatment for young adults with possible mental illnesses relative to comparison group. *Health Aff* (Millwood). 2014; 33(8): 1425-1434. doi:10.1377/hlthaff.2014.0214.

[97] Busch SH, Epstein AJ, Harhay MO, et al. The effects of federal parity on substance use disorder treatment. *Am J Manag Care*. 2014; 20(1): 76-82.

[98] Centers for Medicare & Medicaid Services (CMS). *Medicaid and Children's Health Insurance Programs; Mental Health Parity and Addiction Equity Act of 2008; the Application of Mental Health Parity Requirements to Coverage Offered by Medicaid Managed Care Organizations, the Children's Health Insurance Program (CHIP), and Alternative Benefit Plans*. 81 FR 18389. 42 CFR 438, 440, 456, 457. March 30, 2016. https://www.federalregister.gov/documents/2016/03/30/2016-06876/medicaid-and-childrens-health-insurance-programs-mental-health-parity-and-addiction-equity-act-of. Accessed September 21, 2017.

[99] National Committee for Quality Assurance (NCQA). *Technical Specifications for Health Plans*. Washington, DC: NCQA; 2015.

[100] National Quality Forum (NQF). *About Us*. NQF website; 2017. http://www.qualityforum.org/About_NQF/. Accessed September 21, 2017.

[101] Garnick DW, Lee MT, Horgan C, et al. Lessons from five states: Public sector use of the Washington Circle performance measures. *J Subst Abuse Treat*. 2011; 40(3): 241-254. doi:10.1016/j.jsat.2010.11.008.

[102] Garnick DW, Horgan CM, Chalk M. Performance measures for alcohol and other drug services. *Alcohol Res Health*. 2006; 29(1): 19-26.

[103] National Committee for Quality Assurance (NCQA). *HEDIS® and Performance Measurement: Measuring Performance*. NCQA website; 2017. http://www.ncqa.org/hedis-quality-measurement. Accessed September 21, 2017.

[104] National Quality Forum (NQF). *Initiation and Engagement of Alcohol and Other Drug Dependence Treatment (IET)*. NQF Web site; 2017. http://www.qualityforum.org/Measures_Reports_Tools.aspx. Accessed September 21, 2017.

[105] Centers for Medicare & Medicaid Services (CMS). *2017 Core Set of Adult Health Care Quality Measures for Medicaid (Adult Core Set)*. CMS website; 2017. https://www.medicaid.gov/medicaid/quality-of-care/downloads/2017-adult-core- set.pdf. Accessed September 21, 2017.

[106] Personal communications from D.E.B. Potter, Staff Co-Chair, U.S. Department of Health and Human Services, Behavioral Health Coordinating Committee, Subcommittee on Quality Measures.

[107] Substance Abuse and Mental Health Services Administration (SAMHSA). Quality Measures. *SAMHSA website*. Last updated April 18, 2017. https://www.samhsa.gov/section-223/quality-measures. Accessed September 21, 2017.

[108] Centers for Medicare & Medicaid Services (CMS). *MIPS Overview*. Quality Payment Program website; 2017. https://qpp.cms.gov/mips/overview. Accessed September 21, 2017.

[109] Zainulbhai S, Goldberg L, Ng W, Montgomery A. Assessing care integration for dual-eligible beneficiaries: A review of quality measures chosen by states in the financial alignment initiative. *Issue Brief* (Commonw Fund). 2014; 2: 1-20.

[110] National Quality Forum (NQF). *Alignment Tool. Measure Applications Partnership (MAP) Duals Eligible Beneficiaries Workgroup.* NQF website. 2015. http://www.qualityforum.org/Calendar/2015/03/MAP_Dual_Eligible_Beneficiaries_In-Person_Meeting_03042015.aspx. Accessed September 21, 2017.

[111] *Center for Health Care Strategies. Quality Measurement Approaches of State Medicaid Accountable Care Organization Programs, Technical Assistance Tool.* Trenton, NJ: Center for Health Care Strategies; 2017. http://www.chcs.org/media/QM_Medicaid- ACOs_matrix050217.pdf. Accessed September 21, 2017.

[112] Harris AHS, Reeder RN, Ellerbe LS, Bowe TR. Validation of the treatment identification strategy of the HEDIS addiction quality measures: Concordance with medical record review. *BMC Health Serv Res*. 2011; 11(1): 73. doi:10.1186/1472-6963-11-73.

[113] Harris AHS, Ellerbe L, Phelps TE, et al. Examining the specification validity of the HEDIS quality measures for substance use disorders. *J Subst Abuse Treat*. 2015; 53: 16-21. doi:10.1016/j.jsat.2015.01.002.

[114] Harris AHS, Humphreys K, Bowe T, Tiet Q, Finney JW. Does meeting the HEDIS substance abuse treatment engagement criterion predict patient outcomes? *J Behav Heal Serv Res*. 2010; 37(1): 25-39. doi:10.1007/s11414-008-9142-2.

[115] Garnick DW, Lee MT, O'Brien PL, et al. The Washington circle engagement performance measures' association with adolescent treatment outcomes. *Drug Alcohol Depend*. 2012; 124(3): 250-258. doi:10.1016/j.drugalcdep.2012.01.011.

[116] Garnick DW, Horgan CM, Acevedo A, et al. Criminal justice outcomes after engagement in outpatient substance abuse treatment. *J Subst Abuse Treat*. 2014; 46(3): 295-305. doi:10.1016/j.jsat.2013.10.005.

[117] Dunigan R, Acevedo A, Campbell K, et al. Engagement in outpatient substance abuse treatment and employment outcomes. *J*

Behav Heal Serv Res. 2014; 41(1): 20-36. doi:10.1007/s11414-013-9334-2.

[118] National Committee for Quality Assurance (NCQA). *Summary Table of Measures, Product Lines and Changes.* HEDIS 2018, Volume 2; 2017. http://www.ncqa.org/Portals/0/HEDISQM/HEDIS 2018/HEDIS 2018 Measures.pdf?ver=2017-06-28-134644-370. Accessed September 21, 2017.

[119] National Committee for Quality Assurance (NCQA). *Quality Compass.* NCQA website. 2015. http://www.ncqa.org/tabid/177/ Default.aspx. Accessed September 21, 2017.

[120] Glasner-Edwards S, Rawson R. Evidence-based practices in addiction treatment: review and recommendations for public policy. *Health Policy*. 2010; 97(2-3): 93-104. doi:10.1016/j.healthpol. 2010.05.013.

[121] Labbe AK, Slaymaker V, Kelly JF. Toward enhancing 12-step facilitation among young people: a systematic qualitative investigation of young adults' 12-step experiences. *Subst Abus*. 2014; 35(4): 399-407. doi:10.1080/08897077.2014.950001.

[122] Kelly JF, Stout RL, Slaymaker V. Emerging adults' treatment outcomes in relation to 12-step mutual-help attendance and active involvement. *Drug Alcohol Depend*. 2013; 129(1-2): 151-157. doi:10.1016/j.drugalcdep.2012.10.005.

[123] Labbe AK, Greene C, Bergman BG, Hoeppner B, Kelly JF. The importance of age composition of 12-step meetings as a moderating factor in the relation between young adults' 12-step participation and abstinence. *Drug Alcohol Depend*. 2013; 133(2): 541-547. doi:10.1016/j.drugalcdep.2013.07.021.

[124] O'Malley SS, Corbin WR, Leeman RF, et al. Reduction of alcohol drinking in young adults by naltrexone: a double-blind, placebo-controlled, randomized clinical trial of efficacy and safety. *J Clin Psychiatry*. 2015; 76(2): e207-e213. doi:10.4088/JCP.13m08934.

[125] Croff RL, Rieckmann TR, Spence JD. Provider and state perspectives on implementing cultural-based models of care for american Indian and alaska native patients with substance use

disorders. *J Behav Health Serv Res*. 2014; 41(1): 64-79. doi:10.1007/s11414-013-9322-6.

[126] Gaudiano BA, Weinstock LM, Miller IW. Improving treatment adherence in bipolar disorder: A review of current psychosocial treatment efficacy and recommendations for future treatment development. *Behav Modif*. 2008; 32(3): 267-301. doi:10.1177/0145445507309023.

[127] Molfenter T. Reducing appointment no-shows: Going from theory to practice. *Subst Use Misuse*. 2013; 48(9): 743-749. doi:10.3109/10826084.2013.787098.

[128] Loveland D, Driscoll H. Examining attrition rates at one specialty addiction treatment provider in the United States: A case study using a retrospective chart review. *Subst Abuse Treat Prev Policy*. 2014; 9(41). doi:10.1186/1747-597X-9-41.

[129] Rutkowski BA, Gallon S, Rawson RA, et al. Improving client engagement and retention in treatment: The Los Angeles County experience. *J Subst Abuse Treat*. 2010; 39(1): 78-86. doi:10.1016/j.jsat.2010.03.015.

[130] Guy R, Hocking J, Wand H, Stott S, Ali H, Kaldor J. How effective are short message service reminders at increasing clinic attendance? A meta-analysis and systematic review. *Health Serv Res*. 2012; 47(2): 614-632. doi:10.1111/j.1475-6773.2011.01342.x.

[131] Gurol-Urganci I, De Jongh T, Atun R, Car J. Mobile phone messaging reminders for attendance at healthcare appointments. *Cochrane Database Syst Rev*. 2012; (7): CD007458. doi:10.1002/14651858.CD007458.pub2.

[132] Hasvold PE, Wootton R. Use of telephone and SMS reminders to improve attendance at hospital appointments: a systematic review. *J Telemed Telecare*. 2011; 17(7): 358-364. doi:10.1258/jtt.2011.110707.

[133] Spohr SA, Taxman FS, Walters ST. The relationship between electronic goal reminders and subsequent drug use and treatment initiation in a criminal justice setting. *Addict Behav*. 2015; 51: 51-56. doi:10.1016/j.addbeh.2015.07.005.

[134] Bradley KA, Kivlahan DR. Bringing patient-centered care to patients with alcohol use disorders. *JAMA*. 2014; 311(18): 1861-1862. doi:10.1001/jama.2014.3629.

[135] Moses K, Klebonis J. *Designing Medicaid health homes for individuals with opioid dependency: Considerations for states.* Health Home Information Resource Center. Baltimore, MD: CMS; 2015. http://www.medicaid.gov/state-resource-center/medicaid-state-technical-assistance/health-homes-technical-assistance/downloads/health-homes-for-opiod-dependency.pdf. Accessed September 21, 2017.

[136] Epstein RM, Fiscella K, Lesser CS, Stange KC. Why the nation needs a policy push on patient-centered health care. *Health Aff* (Millwood). 2010; 29(8): 1489-1495. doi:10.1377/hlthaff.2009.0888.

[137] Légaré F, Witteman HO. Shared decision making: Examining key elements and barriers to adoption into routine clinical practice. *Health Aff* (Millwood). 2013; 32(2): 276-284. doi:10.1377/hlthaff.2012.1078.

[138] Barry MJ, Edgman-Levitan S. Shared decision making – pinnacle of patient-centered care. *N Engl J Med*. 2012; 366(9): 780-781. doi:10.1056/NEJMp1109283.

[139] Miles J, Mericle AA, Way F, Cacciola J. Patient-centered care coordination: A qualitative study of the lived experience of residents in Philadelphia recovery homes. *Addict Sci Clin Pract*. 2015; 10(Suppl 1): A39. doi:10.1186/1940-0640-10-S1-A39.

[140] Xing J, Goehring C, Mancuso D. Care coordination program for Washington state Medicaid enrollees reduced inpatient hospital costs. *Health Aff* (Millwood). 2015; 34(4): 653-661. doi:10.1377/hlthaff.2014.0655.

[141] Brown RS, Peikes D, Peterson G, Schore J, Razafindrakoto CM. Six features of Medicare coordinated care demonstration programs that cut hospital admissions of high-risk patients. *Health Aff* (Millwood). 2012; 31(6): 1156-1166. doi:10.1377/hlthaff.2012.0393.

[142] Healthcare Fraud Prevention Partnership. *Healthcare Payer Strategies to Reduce the Harms of Opioids*. White Paper. Baltimore, MD: CMS; 2017.

[143] Oregon Health Authority (OHA). *Behavioral Health Collaborative Report.* Salem, OR: OHA; 2017. https://olis.leg.state.or.us/liz/2017R1/Downloads/CommitteeMeetingDocument/107590. Accessed September 21, 2017.

[144] California Health Care Foundation. *Case Studies: Three California Health Plans Take Action Against Opioid Overuse.* Oakland, CA: California Health Care Foundation; 2017.

[145] Centers for Medicare & Medicaid Services (CMS). *License Agreements.* CMS website; 2017. https://www.medicaid.gov/license-agreement-cpt- nubc.html?file=%2Fmedicaid%2Fquality-of-care%2Fdownloads%2F2016-adult-value-set-directory.zip. Accessed September 21, 2017.

[146] Substance Abuse and Mental Health Services Administration (SAMHSA), *Center for Behavioral Health Statistics and Quality. 2013-2014 National Survey on Drug Use and Health: Model-Based Prevalence Estimates (50 States and the District of Columbia).* BHSIS Series S-73, HHS Publication No. (SMA) 14-489. Rockville, MD: SAMHSA; 2014.

[147] Centers for Disease Control and Prevention (CDC). *Opioid Painkiller Prescribing Infographic.* CDC website. Atlanta, GA: CDC. Updated July 1, 2014. http://www.cdc.gov/vitalsigns/opioid-prescribing/infographic.html. Accessed April 6, 2016.

[148] Substance Abuse and Mental Health Services Administration (SAMHSA). *National Survey of Substance Abuse Treatment Services (N-SSATS): 2013.* Data on Substance Abuse Treatment Facilities. BHSIS Series S-73, HHS Publication No. (SMA) 14-4890. Rockville, MD: SAMHSA; 2014.

[149] Substance Abuse and Mental Health Services Administration (SAMHSA). *Buprenorphine Treatment Physician Locator.* SAMHSA website. http://www.samhsa.gov/medication- assisted-treatment/physician-program-data/treatment-physician-locator. Accessed April 6, 2016.

[150] U.S. Census Bureau. *2014 Population Estimates*, Data. U.S. Census Bureau website. https://www2.census.gov/programs-surveys/popest/datasets/2010- 2014/national/totals/. Accessed April 6, 2016.

[151] U.S. Census Bureau. *QuickFacts*, United States (2014). U.S. Census Bureau website. http://www.census.gov/quickfacts/table/PST045215/00. Accessed April 6, 2016.

[152] U.S. Census Bureau. *Poverty, Poverty Thresholds* (2014). U.S. Census Bureau website. https://factfinder.census.gov/faces/tableservices/jsf/pages/productview.xhtml?pid=ACS_14_1YR_S1701&prodType=table. Accessed April 6, 2016.

[153] U.S. Census Bureau. *Health Insurance Data* (2014). U.S. Census Bureau website. https://factfinder.census.gov/faces/tableservices/jsf/pages/productview.xhtml?pid=ACS_14_1YR_S2701&prodType=table. Accessed April 6, 2016.

[154] National Alliance for Model State Drug Laws (NAMSDL). 2015 *Annual Review of Prescription Monitoring Programs*. Manchester, IA: NAMSDL; 2015.

[155] Substance Abuse and Mental Health Services Administration (SAMHSA). *Funding and Characteristics of Single State Agencies for Substance Abuse Services and State Mental Health Agencies*, 2013. HHS Publication No. SMA-15-4926. Rockville, MD: SAMHSA; 2015.

[156] Harris KM, Edlund MJ. Use of mental health care and substance abuse treatment among adults with co-occurring disorders. *Psychiatr Serv*. 2005; 56(8): 954-959. doi:10.1176/appi.ps.56.8.954.

[157] Roberts AW, Farley JF, Holmes GM, et al. Controlled substance lock-in programs: Examining an unintended consequence of a prescription drug abuse policy. *Health Aff* (Millwood). 2016; 35(10): 1884-1892. doi:10.1377/hlthaff.2016.0355.

APPENDIX A. GLOSSARY AND ACRONYMS

Table A.1. Glossary of terms and definitions

Term	Definition
Acamprosate	A prescription medication used to aid individuals who are alcohol dependent; approved by the Federal Drug Administration in July 2004 for post-withdrawal maintenance of alcohol abstinence.[a]
Addiction Severity Index (ASI) Alcohol, Drug and Legal Composite Scores	A semi-structured clinical interview used to generate a diagnostic understanding of individuals' substance use treatment needs. The assessment measures need in 7 problem areas including medical, employment/support, alcohol, drug, legal, family/social, and psychiatric. Composite scores from each problem area represent measures of problem severity to generate deeper understanding of treatment planning and evaluation.[b]
Affordable Care Act (Patient Protection and Affordable Care Act and the Health Care and Education Reconciliation Act of 2010)	The Affordable Care Act collectively refers to the Patient Protection and Affordable Care Act and the Health Care and Education Reconciliation Act that were enacted in March 2010. These legislations expanded access to health insurance for lower-income households by establishing subsidies to offset costs of insurance premiums for households with incomes between 100%-400% of the federal poverty level. The legislations also enabled states to expand Medicaid coverage to adults with incomes below 138% of the federal poverty level. Specific to substance use treatment, the Affordable Care Act requires group health plans, group health insurance, and individual health insurance to provide behavioral health care benefits at parity with medical and surgical benefits.[c]
Alcohol use disorder	A pattern of alcohol use that involves problems controlling drinking, being preoccupied with alcohol, continuing to use alcohol even when it causes problems, having to drink more to get the same effect, or having withdrawal symptoms when rapidly decreasing or stopping drinking.[d]
Binge drinking	A pattern of consuming excessive amounts of alcohol in a short period of time. National guidelines define binge drinking as consuming alcohol in a way that brings blood alcohol concentration levels to 0.08g/dL, which is generally translated to 5 drinks for men and 4 drinks for women during a single drinking episode.[e]
Buprenorphine	Buprenorphine is a medication used in the treatment of opioid dependency. Chemically, buprenorphine is a partial opioid agonist and kappa agonist. The dose-response curve observed from buprenorphine use suggests that, although there is potential for misuse, overdose would not result in significant respiratory depression. Clinical trials have demonstrated significant efficacy for treating opioid dependence.[f] Buprenorphine was approved for clinical use in October 2002 by the FDA for its use in MAT.[g]

Term	Definition
Buprenorphine-Naloxone	A combination medication containing both buprenorphine and naloxone that is used in the treatment of opioid dependency. This medication was developed because of the potential for diversion and misuse of mono-buprenorphine formulations. The naloxone part of the compound precipitates withdrawal in individuals who misuse the combined medication via injection. Combined, this medication decreases the likelihood of diversion and misuse of the combination drug product.[f]
Care coordination	The intentional organization of patient care activities between multiple providers, including primary and behavioral health care providers, to facilitate service delivery in consideration of patients' needs and treatment goals. Care coordination is achieved largely through the managed exchange of information across several aspects of care.[h]
Case management	Process by which multiple aspects of an individual's care is managed, including through phases of assessment, treatment planning, care coordination, clinical monitoring, evaluation, and advocacy with the goal of meeting an individual's unique needs.[i]
Cognitive behavioral therapy	A type of psychotherapy used in the treatment of individuals with SUDs and other psychiatric conditions to help them address harmful thought patterns by learning and practicing alternative ways of thinking and behaving that regulate distressing emotions and harmful behavior.[j]
Contingency management	Giving individuals tangible rewards to reinforce positive behaviors such as abstinence or treatment attendance.[k]
Co-occurring	The presence of more than 1 disorder at the same time, which may include co-occurring behavioral health conditions (mental and SUDs) or co-occurring behavioral health and physical health conditions.
Disulfiram	The first medication, approved by the FDA in 1951, to treat chronic alcohol dependence.[l]
DSM-IV	A manual published by the American Psychiatric Association that includes all recognized mental disorders; clinicians and psychiatrists use it to diagnose psychiatric illnesses.[m]
DSM-V	The 2013 update to the American Psychiatric Association's DSM-IV manual that represents the most current version of this classification and diagnostic tool.[n]
Engagement in treatment	Treatment engagement implies continued SUD treatment through additional visits, usually a specified number of encounters occurring within a set time period that may vary depending on the definition. The IET measure defines it generally as "the percentage of members with a diagnosis of AOD dependence who initiated treatment and had 2 or more additional services within 30 days of the initiation visit."[o] Engagement also may be examined under the rubric of "retention" or "completion."
Enhanced outreach	An outreach approach used to engage specific "hard to reach" groups (populations) by using complementary and mutually reinforcing community-based interventions.

Table A.1. (Continued)

Term	Definition
Evidence-based practice	Treatments that have documented evidence supporting their efficacy. This may refer to treatments for SUDs, mental disorders, or physical health conditions.
Harm reduction	Harm reduction is a public health strategy that, among other things, is used for individuals with SUDs for whom abstinence is not feasible. Harm reduction approaches have been effective in reducing morbidity and mortality in those populations.[p]
HEDIS measures	A tool used by health plans to measure performance on dimensions of care and service.
Heavy drinking	Defined for men as 15 drinks or more per week and for women as 8 drinks or more per week.[q]
Illicit drug use	The use of illegal drugs and/or the misuse of prescription medications or household substances.
Initiation of use	The first use of a substance.
Initiation of treatment	Treatment initiation generally indicates that a patient has attended at least 1 treatment or assessment session following his or her identification as someone who needs treatment for alcohol or drug use disorders or following an admissions process. The IET measure defines it generally as "Initiation: the percentage of members who initiate treatment through an inpatient AOD admission, outpatient visit, IOP encounter, or partial hospitalization within 14 days of diagnosis."[r]
Initiation and Engagement of Alcohol and other Drug Dependence Treatment (IET)	IET is a widely used performance measure for which NCQA is the steward. This measure contains separate rates for initiation of treatment and engagement in treatment. It is, among other things, part of the HEDIS measure set for health plans and is endorsed by the National Quality Forum.[s,t]
Inpatient treatment	Inpatient treatment is a type of intensive treatment in which a patient is provided 24-hour care at a hospital where medically supervised detoxification can be incorporated if needed. This treatment may take place in a medical or a psychiatric hospital.
Integrated care	Care integration and integrated treatment is a model that seeks to integrate treatment of physical, mental, and substance use conditions. Integration may focus on treatment, systems of care, and/or financing.
Intensive outpatient (IOP) treatment	IOP treatment is a type of specialized addiction recovery program that provides daily structure and focused treatment activities where a person attends the program on a daily basis that accommodates his or her home and work life.
Medical home model	The medical home model is a care delivery model whereby patients' treatment is coordinated through their primary care provider to ensure they receive the necessary care when and where they need it and in a manner that they can understand.

Term	Definition
Medication-assisted treatment (MAT)	MAT is an evidence-based treatment involving the use of medications with counseling and behavioral therapies to treat either alcohol or OUDs.
Paul Wellstone and Pete Domenici Mental Health Parity and Addiction Equity Act (MHPAEA) of 2008	MHPAEA is a federal law that prevents group health plans and health insurance issuers that provide mental or SUD benefits from imposing less favorable limitations on those benefits than on medical/surgical benefits.
Methadone	Methadone is a medication used in MAT to help people reduce or quit their use of heroin or other opiates such as prescription opioid pain medication.
Naloxone	Naloxone is a medication that blocks or reverses the effects of opioids, including extreme drowsiness, slowed breathing, or loss of consciousness. It is used to treat opioid or narcotic overdoses in emergency situations. It also is used in the compound medication buprenorphine-naloxone. Naloxone was approved by the FDA to prevent overdose by opioids such as heroin, morphine, and oxycodone.[u]
Naltrexone	Naltrexone is a medication used to treat OUD and alcohol use disorder and is available in oral and injectable forms.
Non-medical drug use	The taking of prescription drugs, whether obtained by prescription or otherwise, other than in the manner, for the reasons, or in the time period prescribed. It also includes a person taking a prescription drug that was not prescribed to him or her and is taken for the experience or feeling that the drug causes.
Opioid use disorder (OUD)	A problematic pattern of opioid use leading to clinically significant impairment or distress, as manifested by at least 2 of the following criteria, occurring within a 12-month period: • Taking opioids in larger amounts or over a longer period than was intended. • Having a persistent desire or making unsuccessful efforts to cut down or control opioid use. • Spending a great deal of time in activities necessary to obtain the opioid, use the opioid, or recover from its effects. • Having cravings for or a strong desire or urge to use opioids. • Recurrently using opioids that results in a failure to fulfill major role obligations at work, school, or home. • Continuing to use opioids despite having persistent or recurrent social or interpersonal problems caused or exacerbated by the effects of opioids. • Reducing or giving up important social, occupational, or recreational activities because of opioid use. • Recurrently using opioids in situations in which it is physically hazardous.

Table A.1. (Continued)

Term	Definition
	• Continuing to use opioids despite knowledge of having a persistent or recurrent physical or psychological problem that is likely to have been caused or • exacerbated by the substance.[v]
Opioids (heroin, prescription painkillers, synthetic opioids)	Opioids are a class of drugs that include the illegal drug heroin, synthetic opioids such as fentanyl, and pain relievers available legally by prescription, such as oxycodone (OxyContin®), hydrocodone (Vicodin®), codeine, morphine, and many others.
Out-of-pocket (OOP)	Expenses for medical care that are not reimbursed by insurance. OOP costs include deductibles, co-insurance, and co-payments for covered services plus all costs for services that are not covered.
Outpatient treatment	Outpatient treatment, sometimes called ambulatory care, describes medical care or treatment that does not require an overnight stay in a hospital or medical facility. A visit to a doctor or counselor for assessment or treatment in a non-hospital setting is an example of outpatient treatment.
Overdose	An excessive and dangerous amount of a drug taken intentionally or by accident that results in negative health consequences or death.
Partial hospitalization (PH)	Partial hospitalization provides an intense, structured treatment setting for individuals who have difficulty maintaining current daily routines or who would otherwise require inpatient behavioral health care. It is provided on a daily basis with the person being allowed to reside at home and maintain as much family life and work responsibility as possible. (Also see IOP treatment.)
Pay for performance (P4P)	Initiatives aimed at improving the quality, efficiency, and overall value of health care. These arrangements provide financial incentives to hospitals, physicians, and other health care providers to carry out such improvements and achieve optimal outcomes for patients. Performance typically is assessed using a performance or quality measure.
Performance or quality measurement	A performance or quality measurement is the regular measurement of outcomes, processes, or other indicators that generate reliable data on the effectiveness and efficiency of programs or interventions.
Performance-based contracting	A results-oriented contracting method that focuses on the performance of the contractor to which at least a portion of a contractor's payment may be tied. The contracting parties may be groups consisting of health plan and providers, a state and a health plan, a state and providers, or other entities.
Pharmacotherapy	Pharmacotherapy is the treatment of disease and especially mental illness or SUDs with drugs.[w]

Term	Definition
Prescription Drug Monitoring Program (PDMP)	PDMPs are state-run electronic databases used to track the prescribing and dispensing of controlled prescription drugs to patients. These programs are designed to monitor this information for suspected abuse or diversion (i.e., channeling drugs into illegal use), providing critical information regarding a patient's controlled substance prescription history to prescribers, pharmacists, or other parties that have been permitted access.
Prevalence	The percentage of a population that is affected with a particular disease or condition at a given time.
Recovery support services	Recovery support services are non-clinical services provided to people and families during all stages of recovery and may include social supports, transportation, employment services and training, case management, relapse prevention, housing assistance, child care, peer services, life skills, education, and other support services.[x]
Residential treatment	Residential treatment, also called residential or inpatient rehabilitation, describes either a mental health facility or a drug and/or alcohol or other addiction treatment program that is provided to patients who are in residence (living there 24/7) for a period of time.
Retention	Treatment retention is the level of commitment or engagement in treatment as indicated by a patient's behavior such as number of treatment sessions attended, completion of prescribed interventions, days of sobriety, or participation in recovery activities.
Single State Authority (SSA)	A SSA is a single state agency responsible for coordinating alcohol and drug prevention and treatment activities for the state.[y]
Substance abuse	Prior to the most recent DSM-V edition, the DSM-IV used the term *substance abuse* to describe the overuse of or dependence on a substance such as alcohol or drugs. Refer to the glossary entry for *substance use disorder* for further description.
Substance dependence	Dependence is a term that was used in the DSM-IV but not the DSM-V. The DSM-IV defined dependence as "a maladaptive pattern of substance use leading to clinically significant impairment or distress, as manifested by 3 (or more) of the following, occurring within a 12-month period: Tolerance [defined]…, withdrawal [defined]…. The substance is often taken in larger amounts or over a longer period than was intended. There is a persistent desire or unsuccessful efforts to cut down or control substance use. A great deal of time is spent in activities necessary to obtain the substance, use the substance, or recover from its effects. Important social, occupational, or recreational activities are given up or reduced because of substance use. The substance use is continued despite knowledge of having a persistent or recurrent physical or psychological problem that is likely to have been caused or exacerbated by the substance."[z]

Table A.1. (Continued)

Term	Definition
Substance use disorder (SUD)	A SUD is present when the recurring use of alcohol and/or drugs causes clinically and functionally significant impairment, such as health problems, disability, and failure to meet major responsibilities at work, school, or home. A diagnosis of SUD is based on evidence of impaired control, social impairment, risky use, and pharmacological criteria.[aa]
Washington Circle	The Washington Circle is a group of national experts in substance use policy, research, and performance management who seek to improve the quality and effectiveness of prevention and treatment services through the use of performance measurement systems. The Washington Circle was convened and supported by the Center for Substance Abuse Treatment since 1998 and was joined by the National Institute of Drug Abuse in 2006.[bb] This group was instrumental in developing the measure of IET.
42 Code of Federal Regulations (CFR) Part 2	42 CFR Part 2 was established to restrict the disclosure of medical records describing an individual's diagnosis with a SUD or receipt of substance use treatment. The regulation requires individuals to provide consent to share any records pertaining to services received for SUD treatment.

[a] Center for Substance Abuse Treatment. Acamprosate: A new medication for alcohol use disorders. *Substance Abuse Treatment Advisory*. 2005; 4(1). https://store.samhsa.gov/shin/content/MS974/MS974.pdf.

[b] McLellan AT, Kushner H, Metzger D, et al. The fifth edition of the Addiction Severity Index. *J Subst Abuse Treat*. 1992; 9(3): 199-213. http://www.journalofsubstanceabusetreatment.com/article/0740-5472(92)90062-S/pdf.

[c] Beronio K, Po R, Skopec L, Glied S. Affordable Care Act expands mental health and substance use disorder benefits and federal parity protections for 62 million Americans. Washington, DC: HHS Office of the Assistant Secretary for Planning and Evaluation; 2013. https://aspe.hhs.gov/report/affordable-care-act-expands-mental-health-and-substance-use-disorder-benefits-and-federal-parity-protections-62-million-americans.

[d] Mayo Clinic Staff. Diseases and conditions: Alcohol use disorder. 2015. http://www.mayoclinic.org/diseases-conditions/alcohol-use-disorder/basics/definition/con-20020866.

[e] National Institute on Alcohol Abuse and Alcoholism. Drinking levels defined. https://www.niaaa.nih.gov/alcohol-health/overview-alcohol-consumption/moderate-binge-drinking.

[f] Strain EC, Stoller K, Walsh SL, Bigelow GE. Effects of buprenorphine versus buprenorphine/naloxone tablets in non-dependent opioid abusers. *Psychopharmacology*. 2000; 148(4): 374-383. https://rd.springer.com/article/10.1007/s002130050066.

[g] Substance Abuse and Mental Health Services Administration. Buprenorphine. Updated May 31, 2016. https://www.samhsa.gov/medication-assisted-treatment/treatment/buprenorphine.

[h] McDonald KM, Sundaram V, Bravata DM, et al. Closing the quality gap: A critical analysis of quality improvement strategies (Vol 7: *Care Coordination*). Technical Reviews, No. 9.7. AHRQ Publication No. 04(07)-0051-7. Rockville, MD: Agency for Healthcare Research and Quality; 2007. https://www.ahrq.gov/downloads/pub/evidence/pdf/caregap/caregap.pdf.

[i] Agency for Healthcare Research and Quality. Comparable Effectiveness of Case Management for Adults With Medical Illness and Complex Care Needs. Rockville, MD: Agency for Healthcare Research and Quality; 2011. https://effectivehealthcare.ahrq.gov/topics/case-management/research-protocol/.

[j] American Addiction Centers. Cognitive Behavioral Therapy and Addiction Treatment. http://americanaddictioncenters.org/cognitive-behavioral-therapy/.

[k] National Institute on Drug Abuse. Principles of drug addiction treatment: A research-based guide (Third Edition). Contingency Management Interventions/Motivational Incentives (Alcohol, Stimulants, Opioids, Marijuana, Nicotine). Updated December 2012. https://www.drugabuse.gov/publications/principles-drug-addiction-treatment-research-based-guide-third-edition/evidence-based-approaches-to-drug-addiction- treatment/behavioral-0.

[l] Center for Substance Abuse Treatment. Incorporating alcohol pharmacotherapies into medical practice. Treatment improvement protocol (TIP) series 49. HHS Publication No. (SMA) 09-4380. Rockville, MD; 2009.

[m] American Psychiatric Association. Diagnostic and statistical manual of mental disorders, Fourth Edition, Text Revision. Washington, DC; 2000.

[n] American Psychiatric Association. Diagnostic and statistical manual of mental disorders, Fifth Edition. Washington, DC; 2013.

[o] National Committee for Quality Assurance. HEDIS 2015, Volume 2: Technical Specifications for Health Plans. Washington, DC; October 2014.

[p] Canadian Paediatric Society. Harm reduction: An approach to reducing risky health behaviours in adolescents. *Paediatr Child Health*. 2008; 13(1): 53-56.

[q] Centers for Disease Control and Prevention. Alcohol and public health: Frequently asked questions. Updated June 8, 2017. https://www.cdc.gov/alcohol/faqs.htm.

[r] National Committee for Quality Assurance. HEDIS 2015, Volume 2: Technical Specifications for Health Plans. Washington, DC; 2014.

[s] National Committee for Quality Assurance. HEDIS® and performance measurement: Measuring performance. http://www.ncqa.org/hedis-quality-measurement.

[t] National Quality Forum. Measures, Reports and Tools. http://www.qualityforum.org/Measures_Reports_Tools.aspx.

[u] Substance Abuse and Mental Health Services Administration. Naloxone. March 3, 2016. https://www.samhsa.gov/medication-assisted-treatment/treatment/naloxone.

[v] American Psychiatric Association. Diagnostic and statistical manual of mental disorders. Fifth Edition. Washington, DC; 2013.

[w] Merriam-Webster Dictionary. Pharmacotherapy. https://www.merriam- webster.com/dictionary/pharmacotherapy.

[z] Kaplan, L. The role of recovery support services in recovery-oriented systems of care. HHS Publication No. (SMA) 08-4315. Rockville, MD: Substance Abuse and Mental Health Services Administration; 2008. http://www.pacdaa.org/SiteCollectionDocuments/SAMHSA%20 White%20Paper%20on%20The%20Role%20 of%20Recovery%20Support%20Services.pdf.

[y] Rieckmann T, Abraham A, Zwick J, Rasplica C, McCarty D. A longitudinal study of state strategies and policies to accelerate evidence-based practices in the context of systems transformation. *Health Serv Res*. 2015; 50(4): 1125-1145. doi/10.1111/1475-6773.12273/abstract.

[z] Clinical Tools, Inc. DSM-IV-TR Criteria for Substance Abuse and Substance Dependence. Updated September 11, 2017. https://www.buppractice.com/node/1436.

[aa.] American Psychiatric Association. Diagnostic and statistical manual of mental disorders, Fifth Edition. Washington, DC; 2013.

[bb.] Washington Circle. Performance Measurement for Care of Substance Use Disorders. http://www.washingtoncircle.org/. Accessed September 15, 2017.

Table A.2. Definitions of acronyms and abbreviations

Acronym	Definition
42 CFR Part 2	42nd Confidentiality Regulations Part 2 titled *Confidentiality of Substance Use Disorder Patient Records*
ACO	Accountable Care Organization
AOD	Alcohol and Other Drug
AQC	Alternative Quality Contract
ASAM	American Society of Addiction Medicine
ASPE	HHS Office of the Assistant Secretary for Planning and Evaluation
BCBSMA	Blue Cross Blue Shield of Massachusetts
BHC	Behavioral Health Clinic
CCAE	Truven Health MarketScan® Commercial Claims and Encounters database
CDC	HHS Centers for Disease Control and Prevention
CEO	Chief Executive Officer
CFR	Code of Federal Regulations
CMO	Chief Medical Officer
CMS	HHS Centers for Medicare & Medicaid Services
COO	Chief Operating Officer
DATA 2000	Drug Addiction Treatment Act of 2000
DEA	Drug Enforcement Administration
DSM-IV	Diagnostic and Statistical Manual of Mental Disorders, Fourth Edition
DSM-V	Diagnostic and Statistical Manual of Mental Disorders, Fifth Edition
ED	Emergency Department
EHR	Electronic Health Record
FDA	HHS Food and Drug Administration
HEDIS	Healthcare Effectiveness Data and Information Set
HFPP	Healthcare Fraud Prevention Partnership
HHS	U.S. Department of Health and Human Services
HMO	Health Maintenance Organization
IESD	Index Episode Start Date
IET	Initiation and Engagement of Alcohol and Other Drug Dependence Treatment
IMD	Institutions for mental diseases
IOP	Intensive Outpatient
IP	Inpatient
MAT	Medication-Assisted Treatment
MHPAEA	Paul Wellstone and Pete Domenici Mental Health Parity and Addiction Equity Act of 2008
MIPS	Merit-Based Incentive Payment System
MU	Meaningful Use
N-SSATS	National Survey of Substance Abuse Treatment Services
NCQA	National Committee on Quality Assurance
NDH	Negative Diagnosis History

Acronym	Definition
NIATx	Network for the Improvement of Addiction Treatment
NSDUH	National Survey on Drug Use and Health
OOP	Out-of-Pocket
OP	Outpatient
OTP	Opioid Treatment Program
OUD	Opioid Use Disorder
P4P	Pay For Performance
PCP	Primary Care Physician
PDMP	Prescription Drug Monitoring Program
PH	Partial Hospitalization
PPO	Preferred Provider Organization
SAMHSA	HHS Substance Abuse and Mental Health Services Administration
SBIRT	Screening, Brief Intervention and Referral to Treatment
SSA	Single State Authority
STAR-SI	Strengthening Treatment Access and Retention – State Initiative
SUD	Substance use disorder
VHA	Veterans Health Administration

APPENDIX B. OPIOID, ALCOHOL, AND OTHER SUBSTANCE USE DISORDER DIAGNOSES

Table B.1. OUD diagnoses

Code	Definition
304.00	Opioid dependence – unspecified
304.01	Opioid dependence – continuous
304.02	Opioid dependence – episodic
304.70	Opioid/other dependence – unspecified
304.71	Opioid/other dependence – continuous
304.72	Opioid/other dependence – episodic
305.50	Opioid abuse – unspecified
305.51	Opioid abuse – continuous
305.52	Opioid abuse – episodic

Source: International Classification of Diseases, Ninth Revision, Clinical Modification.

Table B.2. Alcohol and other SUD diagnoses

Code	Definition
291.0	Delirium tremens
291.1	Alcohol amnestic disorder
291.2	Alcohol persistent dementia
291.3	Alcohol psychotic disorder with hallucinations
291.4	Pathologic alcohol intoxication
291.5	Alcohol psychiatric disorder with delusions
291.81	Alcohol withdrawal
291.82	Alcohol induced sleep disorder
291.89	Alcohol mental disorder not elsewhere classified (NEC)
291.9	Alcohol mental disorder not otherwise specified (NOS)
303.00	Acute alcohol intoxication – unspecified
303.01	Acute alcohol intoxication – continuous
303.02	Acute alcohol intoxication – episodic
303.90	Alcohol dependence NEC/NOS – unspecified
303.91	Alcohol dependence NEC/NOS – continuous
303.92	Alcohol dependence NEC/NOS – episodic
304.10	Sedative, hypnotic, or anxiolytic dependence NOS
304.11	Sedative, hypnotic, or anxiolytic dependence – continuous
304.12	Sedative, hypnotic, or anxiolytic dependence – episodic
304.20	Cocaine dependence – unspecified
304.21	Cocaine dependence – continuous
304.22	Cocaine dependence – episodic
304.30	Cannabis dependence – unspecified
304.31	Cannabis dependence – continuous
304.32	Cannabis dependence – episodic
304.40	Amphetamine dependence – continuous
304.41	Amphetamine dependence – episodic
304.42	Amphetamine dependence – unspecified
304.50	Hallucinogen dependence – unspecified
304.51	Hallucinogen dependence – continuous
304.52	Hallucinogen dependence – episodic
304.60	Drug dependence NEC – unspecified
304.61	Drug dependence NEC – continuous
304.62	Drug dependence NEC – episodic
304.80	Combined drug dependence NEC – unspecified
304.81	Combined drug dependence NEC – continuous
304.82	Combined drug dependence NEC – episodic
304.90	Drug dependence NOS – unspecified
304.91	Drug dependence NOS – continuous
304.92	Drug dependence NOS – episodic
305.00	Alcohol abuse – unspecified

Code	Definition
305.01	Alcohol abuse – continuous
305.02	Alcohol abuse – episodic
305.20	Cannabis abuse – unspecified
305.21	Cannabis abuse – continuous
305.22	Cannabis abuse – episodic
305.30	Hallucinogen abuse – unspecified
305.31	Hallucinogen abuse – continuous
305.32	Hallucinogen abuse – episodic
305.40	Sedative, hypnotic, or anxiolytic abuse – NOS
305.41	Sedative, hypnotic, or anxiolytic abuse – continuous
305.42	Sedative, hypnotic, or anxiolytic abuse – episodic
305.60	Cocaine abuse – unspecified
305.61	Cocaine abuse – continuous
305.62	Cocaine abuse – episodic
305.70	Amphetamine abuse – unspecified
305.71	Amphetamine abuse – continuous
305.72	Amphetamine abuse – episodic
305.80	Antidepressant abuse – unspecified
305.81	Antidepressant abuse – continuous
305.82	Antidepressant abuse – episodic
305.90	Drug abuse NEC – unspecified
305.91	Drug abuse NEC – continuous
305.92	Drug abuse NEC – episodic
535.30	Alcoholic gastritis without hemorrhage
535.31	Alcoholic gastritis with hemorrhage
571.1	Acute alcoholic hepatitis

Source: International Classification of Diseases, Ninth Revision, Clinical Modification.

APPENDIX C. ALGORITHM FOR IDENTIFYING MEMBERS WITH ALCOHOL OR OTHER SUBSTANCE USE DISORDERS

Table C.1. Algorithm for identifying members with alcohol or other SUDs

Measure Component	Algorithm
Numerator	The number of beneficiaries with at least 1 of the following 3 criteria: • A medical claim (i.e., a non-radiological and a non-laboratory claim) with a diagnosis of alcohol or other drug use in any position. Please see Appendix B for diagnoses and diagnostic categories.

Table C.1. (Continued)

Measure Component	Algorithm
	• A prescription claim for buprenorphine/naloxone; XR-naltrexone; naltrexone; acomprosate; or disulfiram. • A prescription claim for oral sublingual buprenorphine. Injectable, transdermal, and oral buccal buprenorphine are not included because they are indicated for pain instead of SUDs.
Denominator	Beneficiary-years is calculated by summing the months of enrollment for all beneficiaries and dividing by 12.

APPENDIX D. SITE VISIT DISCUSSION GUIDE

Overview

Purpose

This Site Visit Discussion Guide is for use in the research study, Identifying Best Practices and Barriers to Engaging People with Substance Use Disorders (SUD) in Treatment. This study is being funded by ASPE.

The purpose of this Site Visit Protocol is to establish a semi-structured discussion guide that will be used when interviewing health plans about their successes and challenges in improving beneficiaries' ability to initiate and engage in SUD treatment. In addition, the protocol will be used to organize background information about the health plan.

How to Use

The initial Logistics section of this Site Visit Protocol is a template that will be tailored to each of the six site visits conducted. Tailored Site Visit Protocols will include logistics specific to the site visit including an agenda for the visit and contact information for the interviewees and research team.

The Discussion Guide included in this resource provides both a quick reference checklist of the key topics to be discussed and the discussion guide by topic. The research team anticipates that the guide will be modified for each health plan to include specific health plan profile and background information. The research team will decide which topics will be covered for each meeting arranged during the site visit. The interviewer can use the checklist to ensure that major topics have been covered during the site visit. The Discussion Guide will be used to provide primary and probing questions for each topic area. Additionally, the team anticipates that the guide will be modified using lessons learned or new focal areas discovered as a result of conducting the site visits. Any changes to the guide will be discussed with, reviewed, and approved by ASPE prior to implementation in subsequent site visits.

The Health Plan Background section is another template document that will be tailored to each of the six site visits conducted using information gathered about the health plan prior to the site visit. This section provides useful background information on the health plan and the marketplace in which it is operating.

Table D.2 offers a brief eight-step overview of the interviewer and note-taking process that the researchers will review prior to each site visit. Finally, Table D.3 is the physical note template that the researchers will use to document each interview.

Logistics

Table D.1. Site visit agenda

[Health Plan Name] Site Visit Agenda		
Date and Time	Task	Location
	Day One: MONTH DD, YYYY	
HH:HH a.m.–HH:HH p.m.	Meet and Greet: NAMES	
HH:HH a.m.–HH:HH p.m.	Meeting: NAMES Topics:	
HH:HH a.m.–HH:HH p.m.	Tour: NAMES Topics:	
HH:HH a.m.–HH:HH p.m.	Lunch [NAMES]	
HH:HH a.m.–HH:HH p.m.	Meeting: NAMES Topics:	

Table D.1. (Continued)

[Health Plan Name] Site Visit Agenda		
Date and Time	Task	Location
HH:HH a.m.–HH:HH p.m.	Meeting: NAMES Topics:	
HH:HH a.m.–HH:HH p.m.	Day 1 Wrap-Up Review Day 2 Agenda [NAMES]	
	Day Two: MONTH DD, YYYY	
HH:HH a.m.–HH:HH p.m.	Meet and Greet: NAMES	
HH:HH a.m.–HH:HH p.m.	Meeting: NAMES Topics:	
HH:HH a.m.–HH:HH p.m.	Tour: NAMES Topics:	
HH:HH a.m.–HH:HH p.m.	Lunch [NAMES]	
HH:HH a.m.–HH:HH p.m.	Meeting: NAMES Topics:	
HH:HH a.m.–HH:HH p.m.	Meeting: NAMES Topics:	
HH:HH a.m.–HH:HH p.m.	Day 1 Wrap-Up Review Day 2 Agenda [NAMES]	

Discussion Guide

Key Points Checklists

Purpose

Use these checklists to ensure that all major subtopics are covered during the health plan site visit. Phrasing of questions will be based on questions described in the sections that follow this checklist; this checklist is simply a topic area reminder tool for the interviewers. Each checklist is specified to the interviewee's role.

Health Plan Description:

1) Management structure
2) Location of SUD services
3) Carve-in or carve-out benefits
4) Relationship between physical health, mental health, and SUD benefits
5) Management and oversight of SUD benefits

Benefit Design:

1) Coverage of continuum of care
2) Incorporation of ASAM levels of care
3) Case management or care coordination for individuals with SUD
4) Contracted provider types
5) Coverage of MAT
6) Coverage of support services

Reimbursement Procedures and Rates:

1) Payment types used by the health plan
2) Development of reimbursement rates
3) Impact of reimbursement on access
4) Reimbursement differences for in-network and out-of-network providers
5) Use of any alternative payment models, including incentives

Community and Market Characteristics:

1) Provider availability
2) Regulation of SUD providers
3) SUD billing
4) State and community attitudes toward SUD treatment

Network Adequacy:

1) Measuring and maintaining network adequacy
2) Managing low service availability

Quality Improvement Methods:

1) Quality improvement initiatives
2) Monitoring provider performance
3) Reporting measures

Facilitators and Barriers to Engagement:

1) Facilitators to initiation and engagement
2) Barriers to initiation and engagement

Warm-Up Questions

- Discuss goals of this research. Do you have any additional questions about this project before we get started?
- How long have you been with this health plan?
- What are the major responsibilities in your current position?

Discussion Questions: Health Plan Description

Discussion Goals

To understand the health plan's organizational design and management

Key Points That Need to Be Clarified by Discussion's Close:

- Roles and responsibilities of the health plan's leadership team
- Management and oversight of SUD benefits
- Organization of SUD benefits in relation to other behavioral health and physical health benefits

Key Words: governance, organizational structure, management, decision-making, integration

Health Plan Description Discussion Questions
(If already know answer, use questions to confirm)

- How is your organization structured at a high level?
  PROBES:
  - Do you have any major partners?
  - Do you provide behavioral health benefits or pharmaceutical benefits directly, or do you use a behavioral health carve-out or pharmacy benefit manager?
    - If so, who are they?
    - How are those benefits coordinated with the rest of the organization?
  - What different lines of insurance do you manage (e.g., Medicaid, commercial,) and how do the partners and carve-outs differ?
    - Is your state (or health plan and/or national plan) involved in any SUD care delivery or financing reform changes? If so, how is your health plan involved in those changes?
    - [If Medicaid] What impact does your state Medicaid authority's innovation initiatives have on your plan's care delivery or reimbursement practices?
    - [If Medicaid] What impact has your state Medicaid authority's innovation initiatives had on quality improvement initiatives?

- What is your current management structure, particularly as it relates to behavioral health or SUD services?

PROBES:

- o Who has primary oversight of SUD services?
  - ▪ What type of clinical expertise is included?
- o Who has primary oversight of pharmaceutical services? Do they differ for oral versus injection medications?
- o Who are the other key players and key departments?
- o Where do case management or care coordination services fit in the structure?

- How does your health plan approach the relationship among physical health, mental health, and SUD benefits?

PROBES:

- o Do you have any integration initiatives? If so, please describe?
  - ▪ Care management services to aid members in coordinating benefits?
  - ▪ Office-based MAT (opioid or alcohol) providers?
  - ▪ Co-location of services?
- o Do these differ among plan types?

- How does your health plan approach the development and implementation of new SUD strategies?

PROBES:

- o Are initiatives developed at the national or local level?
- o Who is responsible for implementing these strategies?
- o How is the process monitored?

- Does your health plan have clinical or member advisory committees or similar structures that inform how you approach your SUD benefits?
- Are you noticing any trends among your beneficiary population with SUD needs?

PROBES:

- o Which age groups seem to be more affected than others?
- o Other demographic and geographic trends?
- o Co-occurring needs? [relate back to the integration question]

- Describe your beneficiary population's SUD needs.

PROBES:

- o Do SUD issues lie more in alcohol, opioid or other chemical dependencies?
- o Among opioids, distinguish between prescription misuse or heroin use.

Discussion Questions: Benefit Design

Discussion Goals

To understand the health plan's SUD service benefit design

Key Points That Need to Be Clarified by Discussion's Close:

- Coverage throughout the care continuum
- ASAM levels of care
- Case management services
- Contracting with providers

Key Words: provider type, provider qualifications, benefit array, parity ASAM

Benefit Design Discussion Questions
(If already know answer, use questions to confirm)

- Describe your health plan's SUD treatment benefit array. For each service discussed, who is contracted to provide this service?

PROBES:

- o What types of detoxification services are covered?
- o What types of residential services are covered if any?
- o Are IOP services or partial hospital services covered?
- o Are outpatient medical and counseling services covered?

        - What, if any, are the limits to counselling services? Does your plan require prior authorization, utilization review, medical management activities?
        - Describe the prior authorization/utilization review process for service coverage.
    - Do you have other specialized providers?
        - Pain clinics who can manage members with SUDs?
        - HIV clinics?
    - Which SUD treatment medications do you cover?
        - (*If plan has members in more than one state*) Does it vary by state of residence?
        - Do you require prior authorization for these medications?
            - Describe the prior authorization process for medications.
            - (*If not mentioned*) Describe any precertification requirements for specific services.
        - Do these medications have dosage limits or limits to how long individuals can remain on them?
    - What types of additional crises or support services does your health plan provide?
        - Crises services?
        - Peer counseling?
        - Aftercare services?
        - Case management services?
        - Relapse prevention?
        - Patient activation, family activation or engagement?
    - Do these services differ by health plan type?
- Does your health plan use the ASAM criteria to assess patients and recommend levels of care? If yes, please describe how.

- What case management or care coordination services are available to individuals with SUDs?

PROBES:

  - o What services are provided (i.e., mostly utilization review or prior authorization versus social service linkage)?
    - ▪ Describe the utilization review or prior authorization process.
  - o Are these services provided directly by the health plan or under contract through providers?
  - o Is there any level of integration with physical health?
  - o How do these services assist with transitions in care?
    - ▪ If yes, how?
    - ▪ If no, who assists with transitions of care?

- Describe the types of SUD providers that the health plan contracts with?

PROBES:

  - o Specialized providers?

- How have SUD benefits changed since the implementation of MHPAEA?
- What have been the barriers to providing the SUD services?

PROBES:

  - o How have you attempted to address them?

Discussion Questions: Reimbursement Procedures & Rates

Discussion Goals

To understand how reimbursement procedures for SUD services, care coordination, and recovery support services may be influencing SUD treatment initiation and/or engagement

Key Points That Need to Be Clarified by Discussion's Close:

- Reimbursement rates for SUD services
- Rate setting process and impact on access
- Alternative payment models

Key Words: reimbursement, rate setting, risk, care coordination, cost sharing

Reimbursement & Rate Discussion Questions
(If already know answer, use questions to confirm)

- What is the payment mechanism you use to reimburse different levels of care for substance use treatment services?

PROBES:

- o Is it primarily fee for service?
- o Do you use bundled payments? If so, please describe.
- o Do you use any incentive payments? If so, please describe.
- o Do you use any financial penalties? If so, please describe.
- o Do you use other alternative payment models? If so, please describe.

- Does your payment mechanism differ depending on provider types? How so?

PROBES:

- o Differences for inpatient versus outpatient providers?
- o Differences between psychologists, psychiatrists, PCPs, masters level counselors, peer supports, others?

- How does your reimbursement differ for in-network and out-of-network providers?

PROBES:

- o Are there differences in the amount that providers get reimbursed or in the amount that the plan member has to pay out-of-pocket for services provided by non-preferred providers compared with preferred providers?

- o Which services, if any, are most frequently accessed out of network?

- Do you use any financial mechanisms to ensure smooth transitions of care or care integration?

PROBES:

- o Incentive payments or penalties for providers?

- Describe the process for rate setting?

PROBES:

- o Have your rates changed over time?
- o Do you use a negotiated rate?

- Do you think reimbursement rates impact treatment access and continued engagement?
- Do you think reimbursement rates affect network adequacy; for example, which providers decide to join your network?
- Do you reimburse for naloxone/Narcan®?

PROBES:

- o How is that reimbursement structured for naloxone vs. Narcan vs. Evzio®?
- o Are rebates available to the plan or the beneficiary?
- o Do you reimburse third parties (e.g., family members, others) who purchase naloxone when the beneficiary is the end user?

Discussion Questions: Network Adequacy

Discussion Goals

To understand how network adequacy for substance use treatment services is impacting initiation and/or engagement

Key Points That Need to Be Clarified by Discussion's Close:

- Measuring and maintaining network adequacy
- Managing inadequate service availability

Key Words: adequacy, availability, geographic distribution, wait times

Network Adequacy Discussion Questions
(If already know answer, use questions to confirm)

- Describe your health plan's process for measuring and maintaining network adequacy?

PROBES:

  - o What standards are you currently required to follow as a result of state, federal, or accreditation guidelines?
  - o Do you use time and distance criteria?
  - o Do you use wait times?
  - o Are you using provider-to-member ratios?
  - o Do your requirements change by geography?

- Main challenges to developing network adequacy?

PROBES:

  - o Geographic challenges?
  - o Provider availability?

- How does your health plan manage a lack of SUD service availability?

PROBES:

  - o Is the plan working with providers to develop any new, specialized services?
  - o How frequently does the plan re-examine reimbursement rates?
  - o Has the plan undertaken any initiatives to expand SUD treatment services to primary care sites?

- o Is the plan implementing or considering the use of telehealth or other mobile enhancements?
  - ▪ Describe how your team is using telehealth. For which services?
  - ▪ When did this start and what percent of your SUD population is utilizing this service?
  - ▪ Are providers required to have any kind of specialized training to receive reimbursement for this service?
  - ▪ What barriers do you think exist to offering telehealth?

- Do you think provider wait times are affecting members' treatment initiation or continued engagement in care?

PROBES:

- o What is the average wait time for the first SUD appointment?

- What is your health plan's experience with out-of-network providers?

PROBES:

- o Are you experiencing any out of state treatment center solicitation of beneficiaries?
- o Are there limitations on the types of SUD services that beneficiaries can access out of network?
- o What costs do beneficiaries face when out-of-network providers are utilized?
- o Are there any OUD services that are only available out of network?

Discussion Questions: Quality Improvement Methods

Discussion Goals

To understand how the health plan is monitoring provider performance and what kinds of improvement initiatives exist to increase substance use treatment initiation and/or engagement

Key Points That Need to Be Clarified by Discussion's Close:

- Quality improvement initiatives
- Process for monitoring provider performance
- Reporting measures

Key Words: provider performance, quality measures, penetration rates, utilization review,
P4P, data monitoring

Quality Improvement Discussion Questions
(If already know answer, use questions to confirm)

- How are new SUD quality improvement initiatives developed for your health plan?

PROBES:

- o Are they developed at the national, regional, or local level?
- o Are they implemented at the national, regional, or local level?
- o How is the process monitored?

- What types of quality improvement initiatives has your health plan utilized to improve SUD services and SUD service engagement?

PROBES:

- o Provider education?
- o Transitions in care? Warm hand-offs, case management, care coordination?
- o Pharmaceutical data monitoring to identify high-risk members?
- o Improving members' access to MAT?
- o P4P or other value-based purchasing?
- o Follow-up programs for individuals who drop out of treatment?
- o Recovery support services?

- Do you have any initiatives to engage groups of people who have been traditionally hard to engage?

- What are some of the main challenges you have encountered with your quality improvement efforts?
- How does your health plan monitor performance?

PROBES:

  - o Do you use performance metrics? What are they?
  - o Do you use quality measures? Which ones?
    - ▪ The IET Measure?
  - o What member satisfaction or experience of care measures do you use?
  - o Do you monitor any of the following?
    - ▪ Penetration rates
    - ▪ Outcomes of utilization review
    - ▪ Member outcomes
    - ▪ Successful or non-successful care transitions
    - ▪ Any pharmaceutical data monitoring for maintenance of MAT?

- What is your health plan's measurement reporting process?

PROBES:

  - o Are you reporting results publicly and/or privately?
  - o Do you look at measures at a provider level? If so, do you share it with providers?

Discussion Questions: Community & Market Characteristics

Discussion Goals

To understand how community and market factors including attitudes toward SUDs, provider availability, billing proficiency, and support services are affecting treatment initiation and/or engagement

Key Points That Need to Be Clarified by Discussion's Close:

- Provider availability in the market area
- SUD billing proficiency
- Attitudes toward SUD treatment
- State support/funding for recovery support services

Key Words: provider availability, billing, stigma, housing, social services, state funding, state regulation, community attitudes

Community and Market Discussion Questions
(If already know answer, use questions to confirm)

- Describe the provider availability in the community for SUD services (note for the community overall versus the health plan's specific network).

PROBES:
  - o Residential service providers?
  - o MAT providers?
  - o IOP or partial hospital providers?
  - o SUD specialty service providers?
  - o Peer support services?
  - o Housing and social services?
  - o Community mental health centers, federally qualified health centers?
- In your areas, how much experience do SUD treatment providers have at billing services to insurance versus using grant funding?
- What are the attitudes toward SUDs and SUD treatment by various members of your community?

PROBES:

- o Does your community approach SUDs as a chronic condition using a chronic care model or as an acute condition using an acute care model?
- o What are local attitudes toward MAT versus abstinence treatment?
- o How have these attitudes affected availability of substance use treatment, if at all?
- o What are the attitudes of law enforcement or criminal justice toward SUD treatment?

- How are SUD providers generally regulated and funded in your state or community?

PROBES:

- o Residential services?
- o SUD specialty services?
- o MAT services?

- What kinds of recovery support services are provided by the state or community to individuals with SUDs?

PROBES:

- o Is the state addressing housing and/or social services for this population?
    - ▪ From a housing first approach?
- o How are these services funded?

- Is the state tracking treatment initiation and engagement rates for individuals receiving these services?

Discussion Questions: Facilitators and Barriers to Engagement

Discussion Goals

To understand what key informants feel are the primary facilitators and barriers to initiating and/or engaging in SUD treatment services

Key Points That Need to Be Clarified by Discussion's Close:

- Primary facilitators of initiation and engagement
- Primary barriers of initiation and engagement

Key Words: member characteristics, service availability, specialty services, stigma, evidence-based treatments, chronic care model

Facilitators and Barriers Discussion Questions
(If already know answer, use questions to confirm)

- What are the main factors that you see that facilitate engagement in treatment for individuals with SUDs?

PROBES:

  - o Member characteristics such as sex, age, comorbid conditions, type of substance used?
  - o Geographic characteristics?
  - o Provider availability?
  - o Provider attitude and culture?
  - o Transition in care programs?
  - o MAT utilization and availability?
  - o Reimbursement?
  - o Specialized services such as specialized pain clinics?

- What do you see as the main barriers to treatment engagement in SUD services in your health plan or community?

PROBES:

Stigma?

  - o Geography or local culture?
  - o Provider culture?
  - o Lack of evidence-based treatments in practice?
  - o Poor transitions of care?
  - o Focus on acute care episodes versus chronic care?
  - o Housing and social services?
  - o Logistical barriers (e.g., transportation, child care, translation)?

- What kind of initiatives is your health plan implementing to reduce the barriers described above?
- Are there any barriers not mentioned above that are specific to MAT?

PROBES:

  - o Administrative issues around MAT?
  - o Prior authorizations? (If so, please describe that process.)
  - o Issues working with multiple insurance companies to cover the different services required for effective treatment with MAT?
  - o Adequate access and provider availability?

- Does your health plan have any initiatives to improve access to MAT?

Discussion Questions: The Initiation and Engagement of Alcohol and Other Drug Dependence Treatment (IET) Measure

Discussion Goals

To understand what key informants feel are deficits in how the IET measure captures initiation and engagement

Key Points That Need to Be Clarified by Discussion's Close:

- Primary problems with measurement using the current IET measure

Key Words: MAT, data, coding

The IET Measure Discussion Questions
(If already know answer, use questions to confirm)

- Can you identify any problems with how the IET measure does or does not capture initiation and engagement in SUD treatment?

PROBES:

- o MAT not included?
- o Data access for all forms of treatment (e.g., residential) or all providers?
- o Impediments to coding by primary care providers for behavioral health or vice versa?
- o Other issues?

Health Plan Profile/Background: NAME OF PLAN

Health Plan Overview

Summary

Performance on NCQA metrics

Provider Network

Marketplace and Environment

Summary (including location)

Largest Employers

Leading Health Plans

Largest Healthcare Providers

State Demographics Snapshot from State Variables

[Insert tables for demographics]

Health Plan in the News

[Insert news clippings and summaries of recent and noteworthy headlines]

Table D.2. Interviewer/Notetaking Process

1)	Review Discussion Guide questions and health plan information, including notes from preliminary outreach calls with the health plan and interviewee background prior to the interview.
2)	The lead interviewer and notetaker will pre-select key discussion topics based on the

Table D.2. (Continued)

3)	interviewee's position. They will designate pre-determined timing for each topic area based on interviewee's position and keep track of time to assure coverage of all key topics.
4)	Inform the interviewee that specific respondents will not be revealed to ASPE. No interviewees or health plans will be identified by name in any reports or publications. Information gained from the interviewee will be aggregated with data from other health plan interviews for any reporting.
5)	Provide a project overview (e.g., major goals) and an overview of the topics that will be covered during the interview.
6)	Ask warm-up questions to start the interview and create a comfortable environment with the interviewee.
7)	Conduct interview.
8)	Close interview by asking, "Is there anything else you would like to share?"
9)	Review notes at the end of the interview day to fill in any gaps and record impressions and other useful observations.

Table D.3. Template for site visit notes

Interview Information	
Date and time	MM/DD/YYYY, HH:MM a.m./p.m.
Interviewer's name	
Note-taker's name	
Participant Information	
Health plan name	
Health plan's location (general region)	
Interviewee(s) Name(s) and titles	
Participant Types	
Executives (i.e., CEO, CMO, COO)	[# interviewed]
Managers (i.e., Directors of Quality, Behavioral Health, Contracting, Care Management)	[# interviewed]
Affiliated case managers	[# interviewed]
Key providers	[describe role, # interviewed]
Other stakeholders	[describe role, # interviewed]
Topics covered in interview [cross out any topics not covered]	• Topic 1 • Topic 2 • Topic 3 • Topic 4
Discussion	
[hand written notes section]	

APPENDIX E. LIST OF NODES USED FOR QUALITATIVE CODING

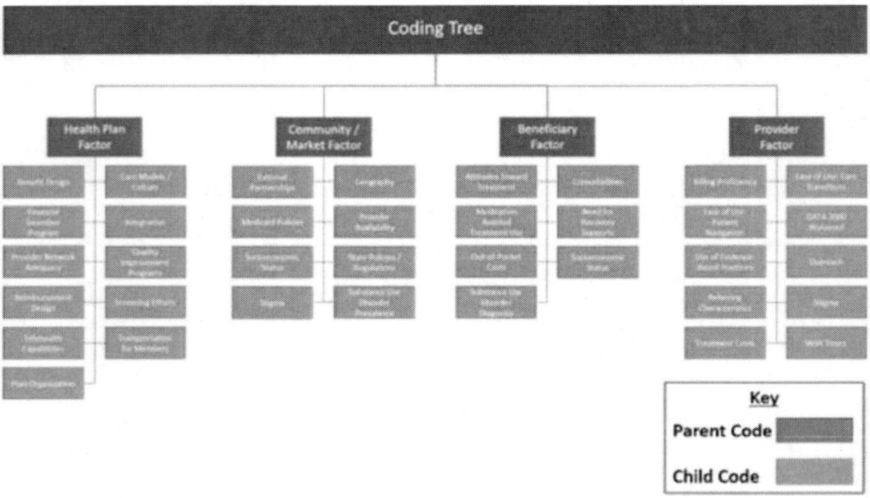

Figure E.1. Coding Tree for Qualitative Coding.

APPENDIX F. DEIDENTIFIED SUMMARIES OF HEALTH PLAN VISITS

Site Visit Debrief: SITE ID 2010

The Truven Health research team conducted a site visit with health plan ID 2010 on February 14, 2017. During the site visit, the research team met with the health plan's systems leaders, quality improvement team members, clinical leaders, and plan-affiliated case managers described in Table F.1.

Table F.1. Site visit interviewees for health plan ID 2010

Type of Interview	Interviewees	No. of People Interviewed
Systems leader interview	Health plan Medical Director Executive Director of the SUD treatment clinic that is owned by the health plan COO of the mental health treatment clinic that contracts with the health plan	3
Quality improvement team interview	Health plan Medical Director Executive Director of the SUD treatment clinic that is owned by the health plan	2
Clinical leader interview	CEO and Medical Director of a major primary care clinic with shared ownership that contracts with the health plan Medical Director of the community health center Executive Director and provider from the women's health center that contracts with the health plan Executive Director of the SUD treatment clinic that is owned by the health center	6
Case management interview	Case Manager from the integrated primary care clinic that has shared ownership with the health plan Case Manager from the women's health clinic that contracts with the health plan Community Health Worker employed by health plan Executive Director of the SUD treatment clinic that is owned by the health plan	4
Clinic tour	Tour with clinic CEO and Medical Director of the integrated primary care clinic that has common ownership with health plan	2

A summary of key findings is included below.

Health Plan Description

The site visit was conducted with a Medicaid plan in the West. The plan operates under a coordinated care model and is managed by a local group of providers. Thus, the health plan primarily serves a smaller regional member population. The plan is focused on providing comprehensive, integrated primary and behavioral health care. It is owned by the partners of a local primary care clinic, who also own and operate a SUD outpatient clinic, and it is contracted with a local women's health center. A local mental health clinic also is considered a delegated entity of the plan. These close associations between physical and behavioral health providers promote integrated care for members of the plan.

The plan includes several committees that govern the plan actions. A quality and compliance committee meets weekly to review member needs and feedback and to discuss any pertinent governance issues arising within the plan. A clinical advisory panel includes plan leadership as well as leaders from health facilities within the community. The panel meets monthly to review changes within the health plan, changes within state Medicaid policy, and community needs. A citizen advisory committee also meets to provide the health plan with feedback on member needs.

Facilitators of IET

All interview groups described their co-located SUD and mental health treatment counselors as a key facilitator to their success with initiating and engaging beneficiaries in SUD services. These counselors are located in the commonly owned integrated primary care office. When providers are alerted a patient's risky substance use behavior or have a patient requesting SUD treatment, the providers are able to bring a counselor into the examination room for an immediate linkage to care. Individuals who do not want to engage in SUD services at an SUD clinic (whether because of stigma or other issues) are able to obtain office-based opioid treatment including buprenorphine and certain counseling services in the primary care office. This option has improved SUD treatment engagement in their beneficiary population.

System leaders and clinical providers also cited their universal SBIRT practices as a "distant second" to co-location but nonetheless a major facilitator to SUD treatment initiation. They described the utility of the SBIRT screening for identifying risky behavior, but highlighted the co-located counselors as the major facilitator of actual initiation.

Interviewees also identified the small and intimate community-setting in which the health plan and its affiliated providers are located and the ability to establish trust between patients and providers as key to engagement in treatment.

Barriers to IET

Major initiation and engagement barriers include waitlists for residential treatment services throughout the region, an inadequate number of inpatient facilities, and few DATA 2000-waivered physicians to prescribe buprenorphine.

Quality Improvement Methods

The plan relies on local governance to design quality improvement initiatives. A quality committee consisting of plan leadership regularly reviews members' needs as well as state Medicaid quality performance metric requirements. The health plan focuses resources on achieving benchmark improvements for the metrics they are financially at risk for by the state Medicaid agency. When the state included a metric for universal SBIRT for SUDs, the plan developed their embedded SUD counselor implementation strategy in their local primary care clinic.

The plan also is actively monitoring state and national trends in SUD treatment and identifying way to implement best practices locally for their population. Previous projects have included educational campaigns, specialized screenings for pregnant women, and the creation of a pregnancy resource specialist position to coordinate care for pregnant women with SUD.

Benefit Design

The health plan reimburses for all benefits included in the state Medicaid benefit array. Reimbursable SUD services include medically monitored and medically supervised detoxification programs, outpatient and IOP treatment, inpatient treatment, and residential treatment. The benefit array also includes MAT medications including methadone and buprenorphine, both of which require prior authorization. Beneficiaries also may receive naloxone free of charge under the plan benefit.

The health plan established an in-house quality committee that is able to approve reimbursement for additional services. Plan affiliated providers can bring individual beneficiary cases before this committee to lobby for a specific service to be covered if the service is outside of the typical benefit design.

Reimbursement

The health plan reimburses most providers under a capitation model. The state Medicaid agency sets rates based on population risk factors, age, and certain comorbidities. The plan representatives said this capitation model helps to reinforce their chronic care model of treatment. The health plan also is required to report on a set of quality health metrics determined by the state Medicaid agency. Universal SBIRT for SUDs is included in the state's quality metrics. The state Medicaid agency places a 4.25 percent withhold on the health plan's total capitated budget. The health plan is eligible to earn back the withhold by achieving its improvement benchmarks on the quality measures. A subcommittee within the health plan is tasked with determining how to use any withhold earnings that the plan receives each year.

The plan refers beneficiaries out-of-network for specialty services and generally reimburses those providers at the standard state Medicaid rate. Care managers and community health workers are salaried employees of the health plan.

Network Adequacy

Several of the health plan representatives expressed concerns over network adequacy for various SUD treatment services. There is a general shortage of local detoxification facilities and available beds in the region's residential treatment programs. The health plan recently decided to support the opening of a local facility that acts as a "sobering center" for individuals requiring a safe environment when the detoxification facilities are unavailable. The plan also is referring members to IOP services when residential treatment beds are unavailable. The plan began using telehealth to reduce the wait time members experience for psychiatry appointments. Additionally, the plan is concerned about the availability of DATA 2000-waivered prescribers in their local geographic region, so the plan is encouraging their affiliated physicians to become waivered.

Market and Beneficiary Characteristics

The health plan serves Medicaid beneficiaries in one designated region of the state, with its covered population being predominantly White and younger adults. Regarding SUDs, the plan has a growing prevalence of prescription opiate and heroin addicted members. However, methamphetamine use is still the most prevalent illicit drug in the region. The majority of members with an SUD also have a comorbid mental disorder.

Site Visit Debrief: SITE ID 2006

The Truven Health research team conducted a site visit with health plan ID 2006 on April 11, 2017. During the site visit, the research team met with the health plan's systems leaders, quality improvement team members, and clinical leaders described in Table F.2.

Table F.2. Site Visit Interviewees for Health Plan ID 2006

Type of Interview	Interviewees	No. of People Interviewed
Systems leader	Vice President of Operations and Execution for Corporate Behavioral Health	1
Quality improvement team	Director of Quality and Compliance for Corporate Behavioral Health Leader of Behavioral Health Team's HEDIS Domain Work group	2
Clinical leaders	National Behavioral Health Medical Director South Regional Medical Director State Behavioral Health Medical Director	3

A summary of key findings is included below.

Health Plan Description

A site visit was conducted with a Medicaid plan located in a Southern state. The plan covers a significant part of the state, including many of the major cities. This local plan is part of a larger national health insurer group and thus is managed both locally and with substantial oversight from the corporate office. Behavioral health initiatives and decisions are initiated at the corporate level to ensure operational and clinical consistency across state plans. The local health plan quality teams are responsible for implementing behavioral health policies and procedures, ensuring compliance with state regulations, and developing initiatives of their own. Leaders of the plan expressed a commitment to having local behavioral health and physical health medical directors operate within their community while communicating closely with the national corporate office and Chief Medical Director.

Facilitators of IET

Clinical leaders acknowledged that health plan case managers play a substantive role in engaging members in care. One of their case managers who is an SUD specialist has joined the clinical staff in weekly rounds meetings, which has improved their ability to assess member risk and recovery progress. Systems leaders also believe that their discharge planning and coordinator program is successful in ensuring follow-up after hospitalization for SUD issues.

Barriers to IET

Clinical leaders acknowledged that a lack of screening for SUD by providers was a significant barrier to getting more people to initiate and engage in treatment. SBIRT currently is not well reimbursed in the state. To alleviate this, the local plan has undertaken its own pilot SBIRT initiative with one provider for children and adolescents, which will hopefully expand to adults and in other settings. Additionally, PCPs often do not engage in ongoing conversations about SUD risks with their patients, which is a barrier to patients engaging in care to make behavior changes.

Plan leaders and providers also acknowledged that the state Medicaid benefits for SUD are a major determinant for access to care. Reimbursement by the health plan is limited by the scope of Medicaid coverage within the state, which has not expanded Medicaid. The state's

Medicaid program covers a limited population and does not reimburse for detoxification, residential care, IOP, or partial hospitalization, although it has limited exceptions for pregnant women.

Quality Improvement Methods

Like the overall governance structure, quality improvement decisions and initiatives are largely centralized at the corporate office then implemented by local operational and clinical leadership. The corporate office's government business division approves quality improvement initiatives and utilization management decisions and conducts annual member and provider satisfaction evaluations as well as state and HEDIS measure data analytics. Leaders of the health plan believe that centralized efforts are more efficient and they also view this centralized operation as a way to spread the use of best practices across local plans.

The health plan's Corporate Clinical Quality Management group supports the local plan's quality programs by writing annual quality templates for them to use and to build their local programs. Local quality leaders who report to the health plan medical director are accountable for plan-specific outcomes. However, the corporate behavioral health team also is responsible for HEDIS performance.

The corporate team is planning to launch an incentive program with a pay-for-performance arrangement for SUD providers in 2017. The team is developing a uniform program that will support this plan and metrics for evaluation will be developed. The local plan is involved in a state value-based purchasing initiative, which allows for both incentive and penalty payments.

Benefit Design

The health plan benefit array is identical to the state Medicaid benefit, which lacks a complete SUD care continuum. The state's current Medicaid program will only reimburse for detoxification and residential treatment services for pregnant women. As noted above, the plan coverage currently does not include IOP or partial hospitalization. The health plan employs an SUD specialized case manager to coordinate care for all members.

Suboxone, methadone, and Narcan are covered without prior authorization. Vivitrol requires prior authorization.

Reimbursement

The health plan receives a per member per month rate and is required to spend at least 90 percent of this reimbursement on medical services and no more than 10 percent of it on administrative services. Provider reimbursement rates are defined in provider contracts. Changes such as enhancing services are met with requests for additional reimbursement from providers. Offering incentives or penalties or adding service requirements for providers runs into challenges because of reimbursement rates. All provider incentive programs are developed at the corporate level and local plans can implement them, but providers must accept them. The rate to out-of-network providers depends on the state. Single-case agreements are needed to cover each of the out-of-network providers who are not reimbursed at 100 percent because then there would be no incentive for them to come in-network.

Network Adequacy

Interviewees expressed frustration over a general shortage and underutilization of psychiatrists in SUD service delivery in addition to the inability to reimburse for detoxification and other services not covered by the state Medicaid program. The health plan also expressed frustration over how few local MAT providers were willing to take on Medicaid patients. The state health plan is not engaging in telehealth services that may assist with provider shortages.

The plan conducts annual geo-access assessments to identify gaps in care by ZIP Code. Overall, the plan has saturated the market by contracting with all available SUD providers. Nonetheless, more SUD providers are needed to meet plan needs.

Market and Beneficiary Characteristics

The health plan covers a large area in a diverse state with large urban areas and rural areas that differ greatly. The largest industries are tourism, agriculture, health care, and aerospace. The substances most commonly seen in treatment are alcohol, heroin, and crack cocaine. Young people also are presenting because of synthetic marijuana and bath salt use. Prescription opioid use is more limited as the state responded to the initial prescription problem earlier than many other states. Use of PDMPs and plan restrictions on pill quantity and number of prescriptions has curtailed prescription opioid analgesic use.

Site Visit Debrief: SITE ID 2003

The Truven Health research team conducted site visit interviews with health plan ID 2003 between April 27, 2017 and April 27, 2017. During the site visit, the research team met with the health plan's systems leaders, behavioral health team, and provider contracting and plan product development team described in Table F.3.

Table F.3. Site visit interviewees for health plan ID 2003

Type of Interview	Interviewees	No. of People Interviewed
Systems leaders	President of Public Plans Chief Medical Officer of Public Plans Vice President of Finance, Network and Business Performance of Public Plans Vice President of Care Management of Public Plans Vice President of Community Relations and Product Management for Public Plans	5
Behavioral health team	Behavioral Health Medical Director for Public Plans Director of Behavioral Health for Public Plans Manager of Integrated Care Management for Public Plans	3
Provider contracting and plan product	Director of Provider Contracting for Public Plans Product Manager for Public Plans	2

A summary of key findings is included below.

Health Plan Description

This site visit was conducted with a Medicaid plan located in a New England state. This Medicaid managed care plan (MCO) plan is a part of a larger health plan enterprise consisting of three primary business lines including general commercial products, senior-focused products, and public plan products. The plan's Medicaid MCO falls under its public plan product line. As one of the state's six MCOs, this plan covers approximately 230,000 lives across all but one small region of the state.

The public plan's business line is governed by a public plans-specific leadership rather than overarching leadership at the enterprise level. The public plans business also has its own behavioral health and care management teams that provide services and direction for the Medicaid MCO.

Facilitators of IET

Interviewees attributed much of their success on the initiation and engagement in SUD treatment measures to the health plan's overall business philosophy. Interviewees described an overarching plan attitude that promotes respect for the plan's beneficiary membership and focuses on addressing the unmet needs of underserved populations. Systems leaders described their approach as taking the "long view" of SUD treatment that starts with identifying individual member needs and continuously providing appropriate supports over time to help them engage. Several interviewees highlighted examples of the health plan's providers reaching out to individual members to address their specific unmet housing-related needs and to provide them with motivation to engage in SUD treatment services.

Recently the state Medicaid authority changed the way beneficiaries affiliate with MCOs. Instead of being able to change MCOs whenever they want, Medicaid beneficiaries now are locked into receiving coverage from one MCO for a full 12 months. This new policy change is viewed as a facilitating mechanism for ensuring care managers can follow-up and monitor the ongoing and long-term treatment needs of the covered population. It also addresses a treatment barrier whereby beneficiaries would be "locked-out" of receipt of opioid prescriptions and would simply change to a plan with which they had no history.

Many of the identified facilitators for beneficiary initiation and engagement in SUD treatment are quality improvement programs that were developed after 2014, the year for which we monitored their performance measures. These additional initiatives are discussed below under "quality improvement."

Barriers to IET

Interviewees considered their delay in learning about member admissions the biggest challenge to engaging them effectively in subsequent SUD care. No prior authorization is required when members enter a detoxification facility; therefore, the plan generally does not learn of the clinical episode until the member is discharged or later. Behavioral health team members said that, even when they phone detoxification facilities to inquire about their members, the facility's staff are unwilling to provide any information. Interviewees said that many acute treatment facilities interpret state and federal health care privacy laws differently and use these laws to avoid engaging with the health plan care managers.

Interviewees also expressed challenges in identifying SUD inpatient and residential facilities that would accept pregnant women. The interviewees reported that providers are uncomfortable treating pregnant women, especially those on MAT. The plan does not engage its providers in any quality improvement or SUD education-focused initiatives because these providers would be overwhelmed. Many of the health plan's contracted providers have large patient volumes and are contracted to provide services to Medicaid beneficiaries under the other five MCOs. Thus, it does not seem possible to ask providers to undertake any new SUD-focused initiatives.

Homelessness is another major barrier to engaging members in treatment. The lack of a stable address serves as a barrier to care managers conducting outreach with these members following hospital admissions.

A general lack of step-down treatment also was identified as a major barrier to keeping members engaged in care after detoxification services.

Although the interviewees felt there is sufficient access to acute treatment, they identified residential treatment and MAT prescribers as major treatment gaps.

Quality Improvement Methods

Since 2014, the year of our data on HEDIS IET measures, the health plan has developed more programmatic ways to encourage initiation and engagement in care. The health plan has focused on hiring more experienced care management staff and on establishing a formal quality improvement process that actively assesses member needs.

Through this process, the plan has developed several initiatives described below.

The health plan employs an SUD navigator whose job it is to serve as a resource to any member with an SUD as well as any family members needing support to ensure they are familiar with their benefits and are aware of which SUD treatment programs are in their area. The health plan also employs master's level behavioral health care managers, medical care managers, and clinical community specialists who will outreach to members in the hospital or in the community. Care managers monitor member admissions and aim to conduct a face-to-face visit with the member before he or she is discharged. Their goal is to serve as a point of continuity as the member graduates through the continuum of SUD care. Interviewees noted that they were unaware of any other Medicaid MCO in the state that provides this predischarge service to its members. Additionally, the health plan employs utilization management staff who not only review service initiation but also monitor member treatment plans to ensure members are accessing services they need.

Weekly meetings bring together the health plan's senior leadership, physicians, care managers, and SUD navigator to discuss individual high-need members. These meetings are used to identify individual cases where the health plan may provide additional support beyond what currently is reimbursed under Medicaid. For example, interviewees described how the plan's resources were used to provide the support one member needed to regain custody of her newborn following her successful completion of an SUD treatment program.

The health plan also recently began encouraging members to use a smartphone application that allows users to have instant access to support groups and online case management services.

Benefit Design

The health plan benefits are dictated by and match those outlined in the state Medicaid authorities' list of covered services. Covered services include detoxification, inpatient, outpatient, IOP, and partial hospitalization services as well as a day treatment program for pregnant mothers. MAT also is a covered benefit for all alcohol-related and opioid-related medications including methadone, buprenorphine/Suboxone, Vivitrol, and acamprosate. Although naloxone is a plan benefit, members must pay a co-pay to receive this medication. Crisis services are provided through the state emergency services program. Any Medicaid beneficiary in the state needing crisis services is guaranteed a full evaluation within 1 hour of request, either in a hospital or community location.

The plan is not using telehealth services to meet its members' SUD needs. Per the plan, the provider community has not been receptive to telehealth technology because they would be paid less than if they just had the client come in for an in-person visit. The plan believes that even rural beneficiaries live within 90 minutes of a behavioral health provider, so geographic access is not a significant barrier in receiving services.

Reimbursement

Contracted providers operate under a fee-for-service payment model. Both in-network and out-of-network providers are reimbursed at generally the same rates as outlined by the state Medicaid authority. The plan will, on a case-by-case basis, contract certain providers for enhanced rates when those providers are deemed to offer a substantive benefit to the health plan. For example, the plan may reimburse providers at 105 percent of the standard state Medicaid rate if those providers are serving an area with low network adequacy or if the providers have become known as "the provider to see" for quality services. The health plan must submit a special request to the state Medicaid authority to contract providers for rates above 105 percent, so such arrangements are not frequently made.

Network Adequacy

The health plan is required by the state to conduct geo-access assessments identifying gaps in care as well as time and distance to providers. The plan is meeting all of its NCQA standards for access. However, interviewees suggested that the defined access standards differ from what their actual member population needs. For example, although the state has contracted with all the existing providers in one of its more rural areas and meets access requirements, the interviewees still felt there are not a sufficient number of providers in this area to meet all the plan's member needs. Interviewees also felt that there is a dearth of step-down services available once members are discharged from detoxification facilities.

Market and Beneficiary Characteristics

This health plan serves Medicaid beneficiaries in all but one small region of the state. The state is geographically diverse with both large urban and rural areas. The largest industries are health care and institutions of higher education. The substance uses that are most commonly seen in treatment are alcohol, heroin, fentanyl, and prescription opioids. The state has made addressing the opioid epidemic a priority issue and has significant legislative support for new and ongoing initiatives related to expanding access to SUD treatment and prevention. First responders including police departments also are highly involved in facilitating access to SUD treatment. However, the interviewees described community stigma as a major hurdle for disseminating SUD prevention and treatment education, but they indicated that it seems to be more pronounced in the affluent, non-Medicaid populations than in the Medicaid population served by this plan.

Site Visit Debrief: SITE ID 9522

The Truven Health research team conducted virtual site visit interviews with health plan ID 9522 on 05/09/2017. During the site visit, the research team met with the health plan's systems leaders, behavioral health team, and quality improvement team staff described in Table F.4.

Table F.4. Site visit interviewees for health plan ID 9522

Type of Interview	Interviewees	No. of People Interviewed
Systems leaders	Behavioral Health Medical Director Director of Plan Operations	2
Behavioral health team	Manager of Behavioral Health Services	1
Quality improvement team	Director of Quality	1

A summary of key findings is included below.

Health Plan Description

This site visit was conducted with a Medicaid plan located in the Midwest. This Medicaid MCO plan operates under a regional name but is a part of a larger health plan enterprise. Much of the regional plan's directions and initiatives are provided or developed at the local level rather than by the corporate office. The behavioral health team reports directly to the local plan's Medical Director and indirectly to the corporate leadership. Corporate leadership acts mostly as a consultant to support the regional plan with quality improvement or behavioral health-related initiatives.

This MCO is one of several serving the state Medicaid population and thus has substantial market competition. However, it represents one of the smaller MCOs with approximately 65,000 covered lives largely concentrated in the state's more urban areas.

Facilitators of IET

Co-location of the regional plan's three case management teams – SUD, physical health, and utilization management – was cited as one of the plan's major facilitators for effectively coordinating services and keeping members engaged in care. All three teams are housed locally and engage in biweekly meetings to discuss members who may need support from one or more of the teams. The behavioral health and utilization management teams also meet regularly to review inpatient cases and plan for discharge. The behavioral health case management team conducts biweekly internal meetings to discuss hard-to-reach members or challenging cases with the Behavioral Health Medical Director. Case managers actively engage in face-to-face meetings with members in the community to identify their needs and follow-up on reasons for missed appointments. Case managers have developed positive relationships with several emergency rooms, which have resulted in emergency room staff reaching out and alerting the health plan that its members are receiving treatment and facilitating in-person meetings in the hospital.

The health plan also compiles provider score cards to monitor PCP performance and access. When physicians are identified as not promoting sufficient access (e.g., restricted office hours, delayed appointments), the health plan conducts private, individual meetings to clarify contract requirements.

Barriers to IET

Competing demands for both physical health and basic necessities, such as housing and transportation, serve as major barriers to engaging in treatment. Although the health plan can provide transportation services to its members, the state does not allow Medicaid members to bring their children in the vehicle. This prevents many parents from engaging in services when they cannot secure day care services. Additionally, poor network adequacy for MAT is viewed as a major barrier to ensuring access to care for members. The health plan is actively reaching out to identify new prescribers or prescribers accepting new patients, but statewide access remains problematic.

Quality Improvement Methods

The health plan actively monitors all members who are admitted for inpatient treatment. They compile an inpatient census list to discuss these cases during case management meetings and to conduct member benchmarking. The plan is using an electronic case management system that allows the behavioral health team to monitor individual patient needs including physical health status and to identify ways to improve care coordination and encourage engagement in treatment. The behavioral health case management and utilization management teams also meet regularly to discuss treatment and discharge plans, ensuring patients receive services to meet all their clinical and recovery support needs.

Benefit Design

Health plan benefits largely mirror the state Medicaid benefit array. The state Medicaid authority does not permit reimbursement for residential treatment programs, so the health plan must refer its members to the county for those services. The plan does provide coverage for other SUD services including outpatient, inpatient, and partial hospitalization services; MAT; and transportation to clinical services. However, prior authorization is required for IOP and partial hospitalization services. The state Medicaid authority permits reimbursement for peer support services for the SSI population, although the health plan currently is not providing these services to its members.

Reimbursement

The health plan is paid a capitated rate for its member population. The state Medicaid authority takes a withhold of 2.5 percent (approximately $3.5-$4 million), giving the plan the opportunity to earn the full rate back on the basis of their performance across 12-14 quality measures; four of these measures are related to SUD, including tobacco. The plan is eligible to earns its full withhold if it meets the high-performance goal and 50 percent if it meets the medium performance-goal, but it earns 0 percent for lower performance. The plan also can earn part of the withhold for improvement rather than just attainment. The plan does not have a set shared savings plan to allocate earnings. Instead it focuses its resources on addressing the measure or performance service area where it performed the poorest.

In-network and out-of-network providers are reimbursed at the state Medicaid rates. In case-by-case situations, the health plan may decide to reimburse providers at an enhanced rate depending on the out-of-network need. An alternative payment methodology, determined by the state, is applied to providers working in low-capacity areas.

Network Adequacy

The state Medicaid authority requires that the MCO achieve network adequacy standards for time and distance to providers. The health plan is having difficulty achieving network adequacy in the state's more rural counties. Generally, there is a shortage of outpatient detoxification providers that results in the health plan's referring its members to inpatient detoxification services. There also is a dearth of buprenorphine prescribers in the state, which poses network adequacy challenges. On a quarterly basis, the behavioral health and provider relations team reach out to all DATA 2000-licensed providers in the state to determine if they can accept new patients. Most prescribers are not accepting new patients.

The plan currently is not using telehealth to augment its network access but is actively looking into expanding into this capability.

Market and Beneficiary Characteristics

The health plan serves a predominately urban and suburban Medicaid population. Several interviewees highlighted socioeconomic challenges of the plan's covered population including transportation needs and homelessness. Drug use in the coverage area mirrors national trends, with high rates of OUDs as well as a steady rate of alcohol use disorders. Interviewees were unable to say whether there was more prescription opioid or heroin use, but indicated that both are present.

Site Visit Debrief: SITE ID 8200

The Truven Health research team conducted site visit interviews with health plan ID 8200 on June 1, 2017. The research team interviewed the health plan's systems leaders, a key leader for behavioral health initiatives, the plan's quality improvement team, and core leaders in case management.

Table F.5. Site visit interviewees for health plan ID 8200

Type of Interview	Interviewees	No. of People Interviewed
Systems leaders	Assistant Director of Regional Mental Health and Chief of the Department of Psychiatry Chief of Addiction Medicine	2
Behavioral health leader	Chief of Addiction Medicine	1
Quality improvement leaders	Program Director Medical Group Physician Managerial Consultant for Quality and Operations Support	3
Case management leaders	Licensed Psychologist (2) Marriage and Family Therapist	3

A summary of key findings is included below.

Health Plan Description

This site visit was conducted with a commercial plan located in the West. This health plan functions as an integrated model, providing both health insurer and medical group services to its covered lives. Thus, the plan is a very physician-led one. This large national plan is organized into distinct regions, each with local oversight and decision-making power for behavioral health and quality improvement initiatives. This federated model enables the plan to adapt to its local population needs.

Facilitators of IET

The health plan implemented universal SUD risk screening in primary care settings, which has enabled it to provide more early intervention services and facilitated initiation in SUD treatment as well. SBIRT prompts were embedded in the plan's electronic medical record to improve use. The health plan also has identified physician champions in each of its medical centers to encourage other providers to screen and refer patients to local addictions and recovery clinics operated by the health plan.

However, the plan did find that providers were overdiagnosing patients, which inappropriately inflated the number of beneficiaries who needed to be engaged in services. The plan created new internal codes that allowed physicians to mark patients as engaging in risky use without designating them as having a diagnosed SUD. Reducing the number of inappropriately diagnosed beneficiaries helped the plan to target resources and improve on the engagement measure.

Each medical practice under the health plan generates a daily "Best Practice Alert" report for each physician in the practice. This chapter contains a list of all patients with SUD diagnoses and a note indicating whether the patient is in treatment, has a referral, or still needs a follow-up from the physician regarding a referral or change of diagnosis. The physician champion uses this list to create a fall-out list of all patients who need follow-up services. The champion then meets with these patients' providers to remind them of the follow-up and other clinical requirements. The health plan also generates provider report cards that rank each physician's performance in providing follow-up services against the performance of other physicians in the medical group.

Immediate access to services was identified as another facilitator of treatment initiation and engagement. Because of the integrated model and service requirements set by the insurer, salaried providers are unable to place any beneficiaries on a waitlist for services. All beneficiaries requesting SUD treatment services must be seen within 2 days. Approximately 25 percent of beneficiaries receive same-day services.

Barriers to IET

Physicians cited lack of new SUD treatment providers joining the field as a major barrier. They are worried that network adequacy is not sufficient to meet beneficiaries' growing demands, especially in rural areas. They are seeing a major shortage of psychiatrists in their network. Sufficient access to residential treatment beds also are a concern for the plan.

The plan provides partial hospitalization and outpatient services through its own medical groups, but must contract with external facilities to provide residential care. Additionally, several providers cited members' stigma about SUD diagnoses as major barriers to engaging in care.

Quality Improvement Methods

The health plan's medical group oversees all quality improvement activities around the HEDIS measures and other SUD treatment initiatives. The plan enables physician practice leaders to implement initiatives specific to their local population needs. The plan has a health services research team and contracted consultants to help identify implementation strategies promoting evidence-based practices. The health plan generally prefers to pilot implementation strategies in one of its practice settings before rolling the strategy out across its entire covered region.

The plan also cited the ability to mine its internal database to identify missed follow-up appointments and other beneficiary trends in service utilization. These trends are then acted upon with interventions designed and implemented by the local physician practice.

Benefit Design

All pharmacy, behavioral health, and SUD treatment benefits are organized by the health plan. There are no prior authorizations for any SUD treatment services. The plan does not have any specified medical necessity criteria for service provision, so all services are available to plan beneficiaries.

The plan delivers SUD treatment services through community addiction and recovery programs that may be organized as any of the following: partial hospitalization, IOP, and outpatient providers. Residential services are contracted with community facilities and provided for 60 days. MAT is available to all plan members. The plan directly provides buprenorphine and naltrexone (oral and injectable) in its community addictions and recovery programs. However, methadone services are provided through contracts with external providers. It was decided that the plan would not dispense methadone directly because of the federal requirements associated with clinic infrastructure. Beneficiaries at risk for overdose can receive two units of naloxone so that they and a family member may carry the medication.

Reimbursement

The health plan operates as a membership organization with a per member per month capitated rate designated for each region. Although providers are affiliated with physician groups, they are contracted as salaried employees of the health plan. Because of its highly integrated model and extensive benefit array, the health plan has little need to contract with out-of-network providers. If the plan does contract with out-of-network providers, it generally reimburse these providers at the state Medicaid rate.

Network Adequacy

Interviewees felt that the health plan currently is meeting the network adequacy needs of its covered population. The state where the plan operates sets maximum mileage and travel time requirements for accessing care, which currently are being met.

Additionally, the health plan has internal requirements to provide 2-day access for urgent care and 14-day access for non-urgent care services. Interviewees said that the plan currently is meeting those requirements, and a substantial portion of urgent care members are seen on the same day as their request.

However, there were worries that the SUD treatment workforce is not growing as quickly as the population's needs. Although the plan is using a substantial amount of telehealth services, its primary impetus was to provide members with more appointment flexibility rather than to solve access issues. Providers can conduct follow-up and brief consultation visits with members via secure video connections. However, the plan is not pushing for more use of these services to increase access in rural areas.

Market and Beneficiary Characteristics

The health plan is the largest HMO in the state and thus serves a geographically and demographically diverse population. The plan region is vast and includes several local medical centers with different provider groups in rural and urban areas. Most plan beneficiaries are employed and the plan contracts as the medical insurer to several city and state government agencies.

Site Visit Debrief: SITE ID 4019

The Truven Health research team conducted site visit interviews with health plan ID 4019 on June 5-6, 2017. As described in Table F.6, the research team interviewed the health plan's systems leaders, a key leader for behavioral health initiatives, the plan's quality improvement team and core leaders in case management.

Table F.6. Site visit interviewees for health plan ID 4019

Type of Interview	Interviewees	No. of People Interviewed
Systems leaders	Plan Presidents (2) Senior Vice President of Operations	3
Behavioral health leader	Chief Medical Officer Medical Director of Behavioral Health Director of Clinical Operations	3
Quality improvement leaders	Director of Population Health Strategies Vice President of Quality Improvement Corporate Director of Quality and Performance Improvement Senior Manager of Quality Improvement Senior Manager of Quality Improvement Strategy	5
Network adequacy leaders	Director of Network Development Manager of Network Development for Behavioral Health Provider Network Development–Behavioral Health Team Lead Senior Vice President of Utilization Management Director of Behavioral Health Utilization Management	5

Type of Interview	Interviewees	No. of People Interviewed
Care coordination leaders	Senior Director of Care Coordination Senior Managers of Care Coordination (2) Manager of Behavioral Health and Care Coordination Manager of Care Coordination Director of Community Care Coordination Behavioral Health Community Care Coordinator Team Leads (2)	8

A summary of key findings is included below.

Health Plan Description

This site visit was conducted with a Medicaid managed care plan located in the Midwest. The plan operates with local state leadership and corporate leadership based out of a neighboring state. The plan has several state Medicaid plans, which prompted them to adopt a philosophy of managed care operationalized by local plan leaders that communicate with the local providers and beneficiaries. Behavioral health care coordination is organized both locally and centrally by the corporate office. The national plan can centrally locate some of its behavioral health efforts (e.g., phone outreach for care coordination) but largely values a "boots on the ground" approach by local providers.

Facilitators of IET

The health plan actively analyzes its internal pharmacy data to identify beneficiaries who exhibit indicators of undiagnosed behavioral health care needs. The corporate office generates a monthly report identifying any members that fill three or more narcotic prescriptions at three or more pharmacies that are written by three or more prescribers. The members identified in this chapter are reviewed for potential member safety concerns. In addition, cases are reviewed if care coordination services are being provided or if a care coordination referral is appropriate for these individuals.

The plan also uses its EHR data to identify when members are admitted for a SUD diagnosis. Behavioral health coordinators can reach out as soon as they get the notification from the facility. Plan-contracted providers also may use their provider portal to refer a member for care coordination services with one click. The health plan care coordination team is notified instantly and conducts outreach to the member.

Care coordinators pointed to the plan's focus on identifying community support services where the members live as a major facilitator to treatment engagement. Because members often will not engage in care that is not provided in their local neighborhoods, finding the right resources nearby is critical to the plan's approach. Plan providers also believe that developing trusting relationships between members and the care coordination team through face-to-face outreach and regular phone calls is critical to successfully engaging members in care. Members might not be ready for treatment at the first outreach, but the care coordination team will persist and regularly follow-up to conduct motivational interviewing that promotes treatment engagement.

Barriers to IET

The health plan identified the timeliness of service use notifications as a major barrier to being able to provide immediate outreach to their members. Such notifications of outpatient service utilization often occur after the 14-day follow-up period, which reduces the plan's ability to conduct outreach and engage the member in care. There has been substantial improvement with this delay, but the issue remains a work in progress. This is of particular concern when members enter detoxification facilities or other facilities familiar with 42 CFR Part II. Staff at inpatient SUD treatment and detoxification facilities often tell the plan's care coordinators that they will not share records or provide notifications of members' admissions because of 42 CFR Part II restrictions. One plan representative indicated that non-specialized facilities are more likely to reach out because they are less familiar with 42 CFR and tend to follow the Health Insurance Portability and Accountability Act (HIPAA) requirement that allows them to communicate with the payer. When asked, the plan representative indicated that the recent changes to 42 CFR do not change matters for health plans and do not improve their ability to coordinate care for members.

Interviewees identified the state's transition from siloed behavioral health services to embracing Medicaid managed care as a major barrier to providers truly understanding how the health plan can help care for their population. They cited provider knowledge of managed care, care coordination, and other outreach services as barriers they are actively addressing with educational efforts and trainings.

Finding accurate contact information for beneficiaries is another barrier to engaging them in care. Many members become unreachable because they frequently change their phone number or address. General stigma around SUDs and members not wanting to be associated with that diagnosis is another barrier to engaging them in care, particularly in standalone facilities.

Quality Improvement Methods

The health plan actively works with subject matter experts and takes advantage of SAMHSA and American Psychiatric Association educational webinars to stay current on evidence-based practices. The health plan has started to approach quality improvement from a population health perspective. It is using the Johns Hopkins ACG® System to stratify and segment its covered lives from the healthiest to the sickest members on the basis of their illness burden. From there, the health plan is able to allocate members to receive specific clinical interventions based on needs. This approach is helping the plan identify the health needs of their moderate-risk or moderately unhealthy members and target them before their risks increase.

Benefit Design

The health plan benefit design is matched to that of the state Medicaid benefit array. Because prior authorization often causes barriers to accessing necessary services, all MATs are provided as covered benefits and do not require prior authorization. Naloxone also is covered under the plan benefit. Peer support services are not included as a state Medicaid benefit and therefore are not offered by the plan. The plan also is not providing telehealth services for any behavioral health care at this time. According to the interviewees, no providers have requested to use these services in rural areas, and the plan is concerned about the privacy requirements and costs associated with providing telehealth.

Reimbursement

The plan receives a capitated per member per month rate and a performance-based withhold dependent on its HEDIS and CAHPS performance. The IET measure is considered a bundled measure in the state, so this Medicaid plan must perform well on both the initiation and engagement aspects of the measure to receive its withhold payout. The measure also is bundled with all other HEDIS measures, and the plan must meet all benchmarks in order to receive the withhold.

Providers are paid fee for service. The health plan reimburses providers at 100 percent of the state Medicaid rate. The plan generally does not contract with out-of-network providers; however, if needed, the plan will use the state Medicaid rate as the baseline negotiation. The state is piloting a value-based payment arrangement with community mental health centers, but the arrangement is not specific to SUD treatment services.

The state budget crisis is having a significant impact on the health plan's ability to reimburse providers. The state owes a substantial sum of back Medicaid reimbursements to the plan, which in turn owes reimbursements to its provider network. Many Medicaid-only providers are unable to stay in business and several have stopped seeing Medicaid patients. The state has also kept the Medicaid reimbursement rate in flux, raising and lowering the rate, because of its budget crisis.

Network Adequacy

Interviewees reported that there are concerns about a shortage of psychiatrists and addiction-certified providers coming into the field to replace the retiring professionals. Executive leadership does not identify a shortage of MAT prescribers, but care coordinators report having a difficult time identifying prescribers willing to accept new patients, particularly in rural areas. SUD treatment services for adolescents and pregnant mothers also are scarce throughout the state. Most of the services targeting special populations are located in urban areas.

Market and Beneficiary Characteristics

The health plan serves Medicaid beneficiaries residing in all regions of the state. Despite growing use of prescription opioid and heroin, alcohol remains the most prevalent substance of misuse and abuse for the plan's membership. Cocaine also is commonly used among the plan's SUD population. Many of these individuals also have co-occurring physical health or mental disorders including schizophrenia.

In: Substance Abuse
Editor: Caroline A. Nilsson
ISBN: 978-1-53617-806-7

Chapter 2

EXAMINING SOBER LIVING HOMES*

Subcommittee on the Constitution and Civil Justice

The Subcommittee met, pursuant to notice, at 9:07 a.m., in Room 2141, Rayburn House Office Building, Hon. Steve King [Chairman of the Subcommittee] presiding.

Present: Representatives King, Handel, Cohen, and Deutch.

Staff present: John Coleman, Counsel; Jake Glancy, Clerk; James Park, Minority Chief Counsel; Matthew Morgan, Minority Professional Staff Member; and Veronica Eligan, Minority Professional Staff Member.

Mr. KING. The Subcommittee on the Constitution and Civil Justice will come to order.

Without objection, the chair is authorized to declare recess of the committee at any time.

We welcome everyone to today's hearing on examining Sober Living Homes, and I now recognize myself for an opening statement. According to the Centers for Disease Control, more than 115 people in the U.S. die after overdosing on opioids every day. In 2017, more than 72,000

* This is an edited, reformatted and augmented version of Hearing Before the Subcommittee on the Constitution and Civil Justice of the Committee on the Judiciary House of Representatives, Publication No. 115–70, dated September 28, 2018.

Americans died from drug overdoses, overall. In addition to the vast number of families who are suffering the loss of a loved one, these numbers are staggering for us, as a Nation. It is clear that we need safe and effective recovery options to com bat this epidemic to ensure that people have the opportunity to get the help they need.

One popular option is known as a sober living home. Sober Living Homes are group homes for recovering addicts or alcoholics in the later stages of treatment that provide a place from them—a place for them to live, while they receive outpatient care.

While sober living houses are modeled in different ways, one common feature is that these homes are located in single-family, generally middle class residential neighborhoods. While a well-run sober living home may provide a suitable environment for recovering individuals to integrate back into the community, some Sober Living Homes, according to testimony submitted to this committee, are either poorly managed, or are run by operators who dangerously exploit their residents, and that is for profit.

For example, Advocates for Responsible Treatment, which submitted a testimony to today's hearing, compiled a list of news articles from across the country. I would like to read a few of these headlines: "Milwaukee Addict Recovery Home Facing Questions After Five Overdose Deaths Since 2017;" "Owner of Drug Recovery Home Caught Selling Heroine and Fentanyl to Residents;" another is "Heroine Bust at Sober Home: Police Find Trove of Stolen Items and Drugs;" another one is "Pennsylvania Heroine Recovery Houses Often are 'Drug Dealer's Dream'" —and that is in quotes. They are just a few of the many headlines provided by—to this committee. But all of them indicate that there is a very real problem that needs to be addressed. Indeed, many local governments have answered the call to regulate Sober Living Homes, but many have been sued under the Fair Housing Act and the Americans With Disabilities Act for doing so.

Today's hearing will examine these laws, the concerns with their application, and proposed legislation that they are seeking to remedy the problem.

I look forward to all of our witness testimony, and I want to thank you in advance for that testimony.

And now I recognize the—I want to say acting—ranking member for today, the gentleman, Mr. Deutch, for his opening statement.

Mr. DEUTCH. Thank you, Mr. Chairman. I appreciate it. But it is a vitally important topic. I have some comments, but out of respect for our members who are here, I will defer.

Mr. KING. Okay, I thank the gentleman. And now I would like to introduce the witnesses. I would like to introduce our first witness, which is Representative Judy Chu from California. And also our second witness is Representative Dana Rohrabacher, also of California.

And you know the rules in this place, I am really confident. And so I would ask you, first, to stand to be sworn in, each of you.

Would you raise your right hand, please?

Do you swear to tell the truth, the whole truth, and nothing but the truth, so help you, God?

Thank you, and let the record reflect that they have responded in the affirmative.

And I now recognize Ms. Chu for her opening statement. Ms. Chu—for her testimony, excuse me.

Testimony of the Hon. Judy Chu, a Representative in Congress from the State of California; and the Hon. Dana Rohrabacher, a Representative in Congress from the State of California

Testimony of Judy Chu

Ms. CHU. Chairman King and Acting Ranking Member Deutch, I want to start by thanking you for inviting me to testify on this important issue which has impacted all of our districts.

I appreciate that this subcommittee is examining the role of Sober Living Homes in our communities and how they contribute to the recovery process for those suffering from addiction.

Sober Living Homes, also known as recovery residences, offer a place to stay for those who have completed treatment and are trying to rebuild their lives. However, the lack of regulation around the operation of these homes is of serious concern, which means that these facilities may be unequipped to handle patients at risk of overdose, or do not employ staff with specialty training.

In the worst cases, some bad actors do not encourage recovery at all, but exploit vulnerable individuals in order to collect insurance payments. This can mean life or death for people like Tyler from my district of Pasadena, California. Tyler died from an overdose after a sober home didn't recognize the symptoms of his overdose, nor did they have Naloxone, the medication that can reverse an overdose on hand. Tyler was only 23 years old.

Unfortunately, this is not an isolated incident. I have heard from advocates in Arizona, Pennsylvania, Missouri, Florida, and Ohio who are concerned for their friends and family members living in unregulated sober living facilities.

I would like to submit for the record a New York Times article from 2015 and a recent report from the Department of Justice outlining abuse and fraud at Sober Living Homes in New York and Florida. These reports describe sober living facilities that lacked access to Naloxone, ordered unnecessary tests on residents to exhaust their insurance benefits, and required residents to relapse and reenter treatment so resident directors could claim some of the Medicaid benefits.

Licensing for recovery residences, or sober living facilities, varies substantially from state to state, and there are facilities in every state that operate without the necessary licenses. Further, oversight of these licenses is minimal.

And so patients and their families struggle to distinguish good actors from bad ones. For some of these individuals, they may not discover that a facility is negligent until it is too late.

And that is why, after hearing about Tyler's death from his friend, Ryan Hampton, a recovery advocate in my district, I worked with the National Alliance for Recovery Residences to craft legislation that would help address this problem without further victimizing the people we are trying to help. As a result, I introduced H.R. 4684, the Ensuring Access to Quality Sober Living Act.

My bill directs the Department of Health and Human Services to develop a set of best practices for residential recovery facilities so that patients, families, and states can distinguish quality sober living facilities from sites that are fraudulent or unequipped to offer appropriate assistance to their residences.

H.R. 4684 requires HHS to disseminate these best practices to each state, and authorizes the agency to provide technical assistance and support to states that wish to adopt or implement these best practices.

In addition, the bill allows states who are struggling to address the opioid crisis and all of its consequences to work with HHS to help set up criteria to designate quality sober living facilities. These benchmarks include common-sense measures like requiring that all fees and charges be explained to residences before they enter a binding agreement; that paid work performed at the facility by the residences be completely voluntary, and not impede the recovery process; and to avoid deaths like Tyler's, the bill requires Naloxone to be available and accessible, and that staff and residences are trained to use it in emergencies.

H.R. 4684 also ensures that individuals looking for a place to stay will not be turned away because they have been prescribed medication-assisted treatment, or MAT, by their physician to help them recovery [sic].

H.R. 4684 provides an alternative to undermining existing civil rights laws by creating a new set of standards so that these facilities are biding by best practices and are not presenting a harm to the surrounding communities.

H.R. 4684 is a bipartisan bill with cosponsors including Congressmembers Mimi Walters, John Lewis, and Greg Walden. It has been endorsed by the National Alliance for Recovery Residences, the

American Psychological Association, and the Orange County Board of Supervisors.

Thank you again for taking the time to hear from us on ways to address this growing crisis.

Mr. KING. We thank the gentlelady from California, and the chair now recognizes the gentleman from California, Mr. Rohrabacher.

Mr. ROHRABACHER. Yes, thank you much, Chairman King, Ranking Member Cohen, and other members of the subcommittee. Thank you for holding this hearing. And before I begin I will note that I have received testimony from dozens of my constituents about this issue and how it affects their lives, and I ask that these statements be included in the hearing record.

Mr. KING. Without objection. [The information follows:]

Mr. ROHRABACHER. I also have letters from several city governments in my district on how they are affected by this problem, and I ask that they too be included in the record.

Mr. KING. Without objection, so ordered. [The information follows:]

TESTIMONY OF DANA ROHRABACHER

Mr. ROHRABACHER. As we are all aware, our country is enduring a crippling opioid epidemic. Many of our fellow citizens of all ages and social statutes are painfully struggling to seek ways to end their dependence on pills that have all too often been legally flooded into our towns and cities and rural communities. I come before you today to discuss the impact that this challenge has had on many suburban communities, including those in my district in Orange County, California.

Our challenge is different than just salvaging the lives of addicts. It seems alcoholics and drug addicts are being recruited throughout our country to seek recovery in the wonderful environment of our Southern California residential neighborhoods. Residential recovery facilities, more commonly known as Sober Living Homes, have proliferated to the point that, in my home town in Costa Mesa, it has been labeled Rehab Riviera. Something is fundamentally wrong with this scenario.

Our Sober Living Homes are not actually homes, but businesses that operate out of single-family homes in residential neighborhoods zoned for families. There are no standards or criminal background checks on those who can operate such a business. A significant number are run by unscrupulous owners and operators who willfully disregard the well-being of the addicts they are supposedly saving, while simultaneously reducing the quality of life in communities where these homes are located.

Under normal circumstances this problem would be addressed by local government. But in this case, federal law shields the bad actors with the protections meant for their clients. Federal law designates recovering addicts and alcoholics as disabled. The Fair Housing Act protects them from discrimination in housing, and its protections have then been extended to the business servicing them. This has an unintended effect: states and local governments have been consistently rebuked by the courts that say laws and ordinances that target these facilities discriminate against the people who are living in the facilities.

Meantime and meanwhile, crooked owners and operators laugh all the way to the bank. They operate for-profit businesses posing as housing providers for the disabled—meaning drug addicts and alcoholics—who are being located in residential neighborhoods. All of this is happening without accountability or oversight.

Indeed, the Government Accountability Office issued a report showing that insurance fraud is rampant among these facilities in these states across the country. Tracking these recovery houses and the problems associated with them is impossible because unlicensed facilities are not registered, nor are they systematically inspected.

In short, there is a distinct lack of local oversight and authority. The situation has proven harmful to local residential communities. And, yes, those who are trying to free themselves from drug and alcohol addiction have also been mistreated by this. They are victims in more ways than one.

Furthermore, the neighborhood impact is alarming. My constituents report increases in criminal activity, disturbances, emergencies, visits—

emergency visits at all hours of the night and day, noise, and filth, and trash, and other issues around these particular homes, but not at the other homes in their neighborhood. The occupants are transient, and they are sheltered for only weeks, if not days. And in fact, there is no time—there is no commitment from these people at all about their community or their neighborhood.

Too many addicts relapse—and sometimes repeatedly they relapse—and illegally obtain drugs. After relapse, the individual often—and after they relapse from their treatment, they have no place else to go, and they end up homeless on our streets. This system, as is designed, to exploit people who desperately need help.

And it is unfair to require residential neighborhoods to bear the burden of shoddy, unregulated recovery by reducing the quality of life and decreasing the home values of the people who live in that neighborhood.

Let's do the right thing and balance the needs of communities and recovering addicts. This hearing is a good start.

I will note that I have introduced legislation that I believe would help fix the problem, not by furthering more government regulation at the federal level, but empowering local and state governments.

H.R. 5724, the Restoring Community Oversight of Sober Living Homes Act, would be the first good step.

I would clarify that nothing in the federal law is protecting—and my bill would clarify that nothing in federal law protecting those with disabilities would prohibit local government from regulating or banning these facilities in residential neighborhoods. For that to work, the bill defines recovery facility in the federal code. And then those residential—those in residential zones are exempt from the definition of "dwelling" for the purpose of protecting under the Fair Housing Act.

Furthermore, my bill would bar federal money from being given to homes that are not licensed by local communities.

Lastly, it would remove the treatment of substance use disorder from the list of essential health benefits for the purpose of insurance. Now, that is a very difficult position for many of my colleagues to take. I understand that. But it would remove the unintended incentive for operators of these treatment centers to encourage patients to relapse and gravely endanger their lives in order to obtain more, and a lucrative insurance coverage.

I would appreciate the opportunity to work with this subcommittee on moving this bill forward so we can provide local government with the tools to help communities and to help addicts who are so poorly served by the status quo.

I thank you again for conducting this hearing. It is a complicated problem. It deserves our attention. And I appreciate your willingness to give this an honest look.

Mr. KING. The chair thanks the gentleman from California for his testimony and the gentlelady from California for her testimony, as well. And, as is the practice of this committee, we appreciate you being here, and you will be dismissed without questions, as standard. And I would invite the other witnesses to be seated. I thank both of you.

[Pause.]

Mr. KING. I see that our witnesses are comfortably seated and familiar with the terrain around you.

First I would say that you recognize that when you speak you turn the light on on your microphone. That will give you—the light will be five minutes. That is four minutes of green light, one minute of amber light, and we will give you a little latitude to conclude your thoughts. We want to hear what those thoughts actually are.

And so, I would like to introduce our witnesses.

And then our first witness is Erik Peterson. He is the mayor pro tem of Huntington Beach, California.

The second witness is Todd Leishman, an attorney with the Best, Best and Krieger—Todd.

And our third witness, Sara Pratt, and—counsel with Relman, Dane and Colfax, PLLC.

And the fourth witness I am going to have to have a little help from Florida.

Mr. Deutch.

Mr. DEUTCH. Thank you, Mr. Chairman. It is my pleasure to welcome my constituent and friend, Palm Beach County State Attorney

Dave Aronberg, to Washington this morning. Dave was born in Miami, attended public schools before going on to graduate with honors from Harvard College and Harvard Law School. He was an assistant attorney general, White House fellow, and we were colleagues together in the Florida State Senate.

In 2010 Mr. Aronberg joined the Florida Attorney General's office as special prosecutor for prescription drug trafficking. As the Attorney General's drug czar, he led an antipill mill initiative that helped clean up the pain clinic industry and reduce the record number of people dying every day from Oxycodone abuse. His work to save lives from drug overdoses continues as a top priority today. He was elected state attorney for the 15th Judicial Circuit in November 2012, re-elected in 2016, where he has led a group of 120 prosecutors and 220 professional staff in 5 offices throughout Palm Beach County. His leadership has led to a significant increase in conviction rates for both felonies and misdemeanors. I have a lot to say, and I intend to finish.

A decrease in the number of juveniles direct-filed into the court, and greatly improved his working relationship with local, state, and federal law enforcement agencies.

And finally, Mr. Chairman, in July 2016 Mr. Aronberg created a sober homes task force that has made more than 55 arrests for patient brokering and insurance fraud in the rehab industry, has led to new Florida laws and regulations that have become the model for other states.

Aronberg's efforts convinced Google to restrict advertisements and improve screening for addiction treatment. And as opioid deaths continue to rise nationally, Palm Beach County experienced a 62 percent decrease in opioid overdose deaths in the first 4 months of 2018, compared to the same period last year.

This committee thanks you for being here with us this morning, Mr. Aronberg, and we look forward to your testimony.

And I thank the chairman for indulging me with that introduction.

Mr. KING. I was expecting a superlative introduction, but it exceeded my expectations. [Laughter.]

Mr. DEUTCH. I thought it might.

Mr. KING. And I now ask the witnesses if you would stand to be sworn in, please, and raise your right hands.

Do you swear that the testimony you are about to give before this committee is the truth, the whole truth, and nothing but the truth, so help you, God?

Thank you, you may be seated—let the record reflect that the witnesses all responded with an affirmative.

And I now, for the beginning testimony, I would like to recognize Mayor Peterson.

Mayor Peterson, for your initial five minutes. Is your microphone on?

TESTIMONY OF ERIK PETERSON, MAYOR PRO TEMPORE, HUNTINGTON BEACH, CALIFORNIA; TODD LEISHMAN, ATTORNEY, BEST, BEST, AND KRIEGER; SARA PRATT, COUNSEL, RELMAN, DANE AND COLFAX, PLLC; AND DAVE ARONBERG, STATE ATTORNEY, 15TH JUDICIAL CIRCUIT, FLORIDA

Testimony of Erik Peterson

Mr. PETERSON. Good morning, esteemed members of the committee and staff. My name is Erik Peterson. I am the mayor pro tem of the great city of Huntington Beach, California. I am here today to attempt to shine a light on the ever-increasing difficulties our city and many other jurisdictions have with addiction recovery housing, sometimes referred to as Sober Living Homes. I would like to start my testimony by reading a statement from a testimony you should have received from a California-based organization called Advocates for Responsible Treatment.

Addiction recovery housing takes many forms, one of which is businesses that provide commercial services to short-term, transient occupants, in permanent residential neighborhoods, where such uses are often prohibited by zonings. A myriad of overlapping federal and state law and case law unintentionally grants excess privileges to these businesses.

Essentially, businesses obtain rights superior to those of other households in the same neighborhoods. Local limits on operations of such businesses are interpreted by the court and the state to be discriminatory, regardless of whether the operations exceed reasonable accommodation or grant more than equal rights of neighboring homeowners. By granting these privileges to operate without distinction or restriction, the courts have failed to note that the houses do not even meet the spirit of ADA, which is to de-institutionalize the disabled and integrate the protected class into the community.

In just the last two years, recovery houses have been identified as a concern in municipalities in over 100 congressional districts. Citizens executing their right of free speech on the issue have been sued by businesses in an attempt to freeze public dialogue. Many municipalities have lost millions fighting lawsuits claiming housing discrimination, to which no disabled individual is party.

Unnecessary litigation drives investigations by the Department of Justice, Housing, and Urban Development. To meet requests of Members of Congress for clarification in 2016, the DOJ and HUD produced a 20-page document which reinstated the issue, but gave no clear guidance.

Congressman Rohrabacher's H.R. 5724, Restoring Community Oversight of Sober Living Homes Act of 2018 is the second bill in two years attempting to clarify local control to come to the Judiciary Committee. The first was proposed by Congressman Issa in September of 2016. We are grateful for the Judiciary Committee moving forward to review this legislation, because this issue will not go away until it is finally addressed by Congress.

Ignoring the issue results in disastrous effects on long-term residential neighborhoods, and fuels an increase of abuse in—of the protected class. Better local and state regulations of recovery housing is very much a matter of life and death.

Ladies and Gentlemen, when I was asked to testify in front of this community [sic], I reached out to my constituents and asked them to submit their stories. I believe you have received many of them. What got me were the stories of the parents of the victims of some of these facilities.

In our city we have houses with multiple overdoses and deaths, and all we can do is send our firefighters in to pick up the pieces. A few Sundays ago, someone forwarded me a program from a funeral they were attending of a 21-year-old lady who died in a recovery home. She was dead for 12 hours before it was reported to the authorities.

The opioid crisis in our country is destroying the basis of our society, which is our families and communities. In an attempt to help or be companionate, we have further placed the burden on our communities and left thousands of people who need help at risk.

The City of Huntington Beach has found that many of our homeless have come from these facilities. Through what is referred to as body brokering, addicts are recruited from around the country and sent to places like Southern California, Florida, and Arizona. After the individual is placed in a home, many recovery companies sign them up for as much public assistance and insurance as possible, and offer bed vouchers for local resident homes. When the money runs out, they curb them. In other words, they kick them to the street, and many have not even received proper recovery.

Over the last year our city has had to help 65 people get home that were stuck.

I thank you again for letting us—for reviewing this legislation. Mr. KING. Thank you, Mayor Pro Tem Peterson. I appreciate your testimony, and the chair now recognizes Mr. Leishman for his testimony.

Mr. Leishman, you are recognized.

Testimony of Todd Leishman

Mr. LEISHMAN. Thank you. Good morning, Mr. Chairman and members of the committee. My name is Todd Leishman. I am an attorney with Best, Best and Krieger. We advise cities throughout the country on issues they face, including questions about Sober Living Homes. But these comments today are my own.

If I can only convey one message to you this morning, it is this: Congress must clarify federal law to make clear that local government may regulate recovery businesses to protect people in recovery.

People in recovery benefit most from living in residential facilities that are small, spread out, and well run. The least intrusive and most effective way to ensure this is through local regulation. If Congress fails to clear the way for local government to protect them, then more people will relapse in the very facilities that are supposed to help them. More residents will be trafficked, abused, and raped. More will overdose, and more will die.

I wish this were hyperbole, but it is not. All of these things are happening in recovery facilities in communities in every congressional district in our Nation, and they are happening in large part because federal law leaves open a radical and, I think, perverse interpretation that insists that local government may not regulate recovery operators at all, even when it is to protect people in reco ery.

Some operators argue that anti-discrimination laws prevent any regulation of their business because they serve disabled people. Recovering addicts are disabled under federal law. So, they say, their recovery business use must be treated for all purposes as if it were a single-family household. Congress needs to close this loophole to allow local government to protect the very social model that recovering addicts need.

You see, before the 1970s, care for recovering addicts was primarily provided in institutional medical settings. In this medical model, people were sent to hospitals to dry out and get clean. Many people ended up in these institutional settings, even though with just basic care they could function well in our community. That fact gave rise to a better alternative: a non-medical social model.

At the heart of the social model is this: we are trying to turn patients into neighbors. But for that to work, they have to be in a neighborhood that is actually residential. They need to live in a setting that closely approximates a residential household in scale and function. They need to be surrounded by neighborhood residents with whom they have opportunities to interact in normal, neighborly ways. And, of course, facilities need to be run responsibly.

In other words, recovering addicts need facilities that are small, spread out, and well run.

The social model does not work when recovering addicts live in large, institutionally-sized dorms, nor does it work when they are surrounded by other recovery facilities, effectively stuck in a recovery cul de sac or campus. Yet, to make more money, many operators increase occupancy, concentrate facilities together, and cut corners to the detriment of recovering residents.

When operators shield themselves from reasonable local regulation, claiming that size, separation, and operational standards don't apply to them because they serve recovering addicts, it is the people in recovery who suffer. With my written testimony I have included scores of examples of what happens when operators evade local regulation. The examples turn the stomach. We heard some of those headlines earlier: operators selling drugs to residents; house managers trading drugs to residents for sex; rapes; resident and house manager overdoses. And that doesn't even get into the human trafficking and fraud problems that are so common.

Local government is in the best position to prevent these abuses. In sum, Congress needs to confirm that local government may reasonably regulate recovery businesses to protect the people they serve. Please make it plain that permissible regulation includes maximum occupancy limits, so that residents get the benefit of living somewhere that is comparable to a typical residential house hold; minimum separation requirements, so that residents get the benefit of living in an actual residential neighborhood, not in a recovery cul de sac or campus, and can have meaningful, normal interactions with neighbors; and minimum operational standards, so that those who care for recovering residents are qualified and accountable, and facilities are safe and well-run.

The social model is—of recovery is good. I think it is vital. And we need to protect it at the local level. Federal law needs to expressly allow that to happen. Thank you.

Mr. KING. Thank you, Mr. Leishman. And the chair now recognizes the gentlelady, Ms. Pratt, for her testimony.

Ms. Pratt, you are recognized.

Ms. PRATT. My apologies. Hear me now?

Testimony of Sara Pratt

Ms. PRATT. I am counsel at the law firm of Relman, Dane and Colfax, here in Washington. I previously served as deputy assistant secretary for enforcement and programs at the Department of Housing and Urban Development's office of fair housing. I retired in 2015 from that position.

My career spans 41 years in fair housing work. I have also worked to enforce state licensing and regulation requirements applied to nursing homes, day cares, and group homes in the State of Kentucky, as well as closing down illegal and unlicensed operations.

I have submitted written testimony for a more detailed discussion of the fair housing issues around sober home operations, and several attachments for the committee's consideration.

As the committee already knows, there is a large body of Fair Housing and Americans With Disabilities Act case law that constrains localities from completely excluding, or from limiting the location of sober homes, and also requires that, in general, they be treated as ordinary residential uses. This is well-established case law—all circuits, all district courts.

But the fact that there are Fair Housing and ADA protections for these group homes that house people with disabilities, including Sober Living Homes does not mean that there cannot be reasonable and legitimate regulation of group homes or sober living environments.

Local governments continue to say we can't—that the Fair Housing Act somehow protects or prevents operations of seriously concerning situations, that the Fair Housing Act protects local governments—sorry, prevents local governments from pursuing bad operators, essentially. And that is just not the case.

Scoundrels often say that they deserve the protection of the law. I have seen it throughout my entire career in fair housing. But there is no reason why a local government should be concerned about liability if it uses legitimate and reasonable regulations to operate, to constrain the operation of Sober Living Homes.

Now, I imagine, even amongst this panel, we might have some discussion about what exactly those criteria might look like to ensure effective operation, to protect residents, to protect neighborhoods. But it is not, in and of itself, a violation of the law to consider a regulation or certification process for Sober Living Homes.

And both the Fair Housing Act and the ADA, I think, are behind those two bedrock civil rights laws that protect the rights of people with disabilities—are also intended to protect them from abuse or neglect, not just from discrimination. But they also recognize that, without these Sober Living Homes, people with addictions, people with heroine addictions, opioid addictions, alcoholism will be out on the streets.

And so the recognition of the process is the balancing between providing protection for residences occupied by people with disabilities, and ensuring that those—the operations that are provided are safe and protected by the police power of state and local jurisdictions.

State and local jurisdictions can use any number of tools to protect the residents of Sober Living Homes and protect their neighbors without amending the Fair Housing Act or the Americans With Disabilities Act.

For example, Congress could encourage development of a national best practices for Sober Living Homes, using input from municipalities, from local organizations, from municipal groups, from disability organizations, and from the Department of Health and Human Services to look for criteria. They even could establish and make recommendations to this joint effort to prepare a local ordinance that would pass scrutiny under the Fair Housing Act and the ADA, but would also meet the needs of local communities. There are models for this approach, including an effort that took place in the 1990s that I saw when I was at HUD then.

It is acceptable under the Fair Housing Act to establish registration or certification programs based on the protection of health and safety, as long as they do not inappropriately burden sober homes or require unreasonable spacing burdens or unreasonable occupancy burdens.

Local law enforcement actions can, obviously, be taken to address criminal activity, and code enforcement can be used to address matters like littering and loud noise and alcohol and drug abuses in the community.

Thanks to the committee for considering these issues.

Mr. KING. Thanks for your testimony, Ms. Pratt. The chair now recognizes Mr. Aronberg for his testimony. And we do not expect it will live up to your introduction. [Laughter.]

Mr. ARONBERG. I just hope he didn't take any of my five minutes. [Laughter.]

Testimony of Dave Aronberg

Mr. ARONBERG. Thank you, Mr. Chairman. Thank you, members of the committee. And Congressman Deutch, thank you very much for your very kind and unnecessary introduction. My name is Dave Aronberg. I am the state attorney for Florida's 15th judicial circuit, which covers all of Palm Beach County.

Because of our tropical climate and long-established drug treatment centers, Palm Beach County has been a destination for individuals with substance use disorder.

[Slide]

Mr. ARONBERG. As you see from the first slide up there, this is the Florida model of drug treatment, where you have someone with substance use disorder—usually it is heroine these days—they will come down to Florida for detox. Insurance will pay for about five days of detox and then about three weeks of inpatient treatment, followed by about four weeks of outpatient care. Three-quarters of the people who come down to Florida—excuse me, three-quarters of the people in recovery in Florida come from elsewhere.

So, since we have so many people from elsewhere, they need a place to stay. And so they live, very often, in a sober home. A sober home is just a house. As you said, Mr. Chairman, there is no treatment there, there is no insurance reimbursement. It is just a group home of people, hopefully in a drug-free, mutually supportive environment.

After the insurance benefits run out from outpatient care, then the hope is that the individuals are sober and can return home.

The charge is about $300 a week, on average, to live in a sober home, paid out of pocket.

In recent years, however, we have had a surge of unscrupulous individuals enrich themselves by exploiting well-intended federal laws to prey on opioid addicts, who are often human-trafficked by marketers, sober homes, and facilities in exchange for illicit benefits such as cash, free rent, transportation, and even drugs themselves. This is the Florida Shuffle, the next slide that will come up here.

[Slide]

Mr. ARONBERG. And you see from that that you have someone with substance use disorder who gets brought down to Florida through a marketer, usually through a free plane ticket, and deceptive marketing. And, by the way, the free plane ticket is illegal. It is a felony in Florida.

Then they go to detox and patient treatment, outpatient care. The money exchanges hands. There is lots of kickbacks. There is patient brokering. This is the corrupted model that you see, from the corrupted providers. And everyone is making money off of this corrupted model, including the rogue labs.

The only bubble there that is not profitable is sobriety. And you have individuals in sober homes, even living for free in some cases, because the sober home doesn't need to charge when they are getting a kickback from an outpatient treatment center, a market, or a lab to send their residents their way.

It is hard enough to remain sober as it is, let alone knowing that your sobriety is going to cost you your free housing and your transportation and your friends, and now you have got to move back home to a snowy climate, live with your parents, and find a job. Good sober homes can improve treatment outcomes. But flophouses masquerading as sober homes only encourage relapse and failure.

Together, the Americans with Disabilities Act and the Fair Housing Act largely prevent the regulation or inspection of these residences. And so it is sadly ironic that the very laws intended to help people with addiction are being misused to shield them—excuse me, are being misused to shield those who would do them harm. In July 2016 our office formed a sober homes task force—and led by my chief assistant, behind me, Al Johnson—to crack down on this fraud and abuse. We have made 55 arrests with 23 convictions so far. We also empaneled a grand jury and created two additional citizens task forces, including members of the recovery industry to recommend legislative changes leading to the 2017 passage of the state law that tightened enforcement and oversight of the drug recovery industry.

The Florida legislature, however, largely avoided the subject of sober homes because of concerns over federal law. Meanwhile, our successful crackdown on rogue sober homes—and we are only talking about the rogue sober homes here—have scattered some of the bad actors to other locations, especially California.

We can't fix this problem alone at the state and local levels. We need the Federal Government to act.

First, my recommendation is to reissue the 2016 joint statement from DOJ and HUD with the proposed question and answer that I provided in my written submission to this committee. This would clarify that local and state governments can set reasonable sober home standards under the ADA and FHA for the protection of the residents in recovery.

Second, there are significant proposals pending before Congress that can make a real difference. There is legislation that would establish model criteria for sober homes and award grants to states that utilize them. There is the CARA 2.0 Act that directs HHS to develop best practices for sober homes. And there is important language that would extend DOJ's jurisdiction to prosecute unlawful kickbacks in the drug treatment and sober home industries.

These measures will save lives with minimal or no financial costs. They will finally address a part of the opioid crisis that has been fueled by a corrupt recycling of addiction.

Thank you for your time here today. [The statement of Mr. Aronberg follows:]

Mr. KING. I thank you, Mr. Aronberg. I appreciate your testimony and all the testimony. The chair will now recognize himself for five minutes of questions.

First I would turn to—I would like to go to Mr. Leishman, primarily, so I could pronounce your name correctly for the first time. And I wanted to explore your thought process on this.

I am hearing some solutions be offered and a different combination of them. And part of our job is to sort those solutions out and maybe come up with some new ideas of our own—which I don't quite expect. But it is just that something has happened within our culture, and this is more or less a fairly recent intensity of this crisis that has gone on for some time. And I never hear anyone talk about how we actually fix that problem that is endemic within our culture. We talk about addressing it when it shows up.

Do you have any recommendations to this committee on how we might look at this big picture for the long term to try to get to where the cultural circumstances that enable the abuse, the drug abuse that we have, how we could address that so that one day we may see our children or grandchildren live in a society that gets it right?

Mr. LEISHMAN. Is your question how can we get at the cause of the opioid crisis?

Mr. KING. Yes.

Mr. LEISHMAN. Well, I usually spend my days dealing with the back end of that problem. But on a personal level, yes, I do. I think that strong families and communities are a bedrock to that.

I also think that over-prescription of opioids in the first place is—lies at the heart of the problem. And I think that is being addressed more now, thankfully.

A number of our city clients were approached by a group that is putting together a class action, or has put together a class action suit against opioid-producing pharmaceutical companies, much like the big tobacco litigation. I don't know if that is going to be effective. I think the culture among the medical profession is starting to change. They are starting to wise up to the danger that they create when they overprescribe.

Other than that——

Mr. KING. Okay. Let me suggest that, first—I know you didn't expect that question, didn't come here to testify to that depth, but I know you have thought about it, and I appreciate that.

I would pose a follow-up question on this—and I think a very important part of that, when you mentioned the families and our neighborhoods—aside from that, which I agree with, then we have employment testing, for example, in many of the states. In Iowa we have employment testing that has been in law for over 20 years and it has never been litigated. It allows the private-sector employer to guarantee a drug-free workplace, and it has worked very, very well. That model works. We never transitioned that into testing in the workforce.

But when I am asked that question, here is my answer, that if I really—going to be the drug czar that had to solve this problem and had to lay out a plan to do that, there is a lot of personal privacy rights that would be in question, and it is delicate to approach that. But I put that little caveat out there and suggest this, that if we tested in the workplace, if we tested in welfare, and if we tested in education, the people left that would be using and abusing drugs would be dealers and stealers whom the law enforcement could address, and we would have a lot smaller universe of people that needed to go into sober homes.

How does that fit with your analysis?

Mr. LEISHMAN. Certainly, if it is proven to be effective in Iowa, I think it could have wider application.

Mr. KING. I thank you. And I would turn to the mayor pro tem, Mr. Peterson. And you have talked about the community, and how the community is developing. Are you comfortable, then, that if Congress enables it so that local government can regulate city, county, state, what levels would that be? How would that emerge in California, in your vision?

Mr. PETERSON. Well, our biggest thing is the bad actors hiding under a good program. So we can't get out there and inspect. And if we had the ability to get into—just know where they are—most of the time we know when the police are called, or the fire, but if we had that ability to regulate them—I mean even foster care is regulated, you can't have so many foster care in a certain neighborhood, but these people can buy three houses in a row and fill them. So having our ability to get out there, we don't have to have code enforcement peeking through windows, we don't have to be, you know, late to the party with the police coming or the fire coming. But we can be a little proactive, and make sure that, one, the facility is doing what they are supposed to do, and——

Mr. KING. Just from—I will interpret this that in that—you would have in California, likely, a layer of regulations—if we went to Mr. Rohrabacher's bill—that would have some state regulations, some county, and some city regulations working in some type of coordination?

Mr. PETERSON. Correct, correct.

Mr. KING. That is how I envision——

Mr. PETERSON. Yes, and I am sure we would be working with the county, because they are basically in charge of health and human services, not the municipality. So work out something where that is distributed more around the county in any type——

Mr. KING. And I would like to quickly turn to Mr. Aronberg and ask you if you had an opportunity to review the two bills that were testified to here by the two Members. And do you endorse either one of them? You have got some other alternatives here that you have offered today.

Mr. ARONBERG. Thank you, Mr. Chairman. Representative—Congresswoman Chu's bill, I think, is very promising. I like the setting of guidelines. And I haven't read the entire bill, but from what I have seen in the synopses, it was very promising.

I had some issues with Congressman Rohrabacher's bill, because I thought that it goes too far. I don't think you need to eliminate substance treatment disorder treatment entirely from the health care laws. I think that would probably lead to more harm than good.

Plus, I think if you eliminate the—if you allow local governments to just ban sober homes, I don't think you are ever going to fix this problem. We are in an unprecedented opioid epidemic and, you know, you can't arrest your way out of it. You need to have legitimate rehab. And there are legitimate sober homes out there that are doing good work. We are trying to get at the part of the industry that has been corrupted. And I think that his bill, in due respect, goes too far.

Mr. KING. We have got some work we can do. I thank you, and each of you witnesses, and the chair now recognizes the ranking member from Tennessee, Mr. Cohen.

Mr. COHEN. Thank you, Mr. Chairman. First I want to follow up on your questions about the bills. Mr. Aronberg said he thought Ms. Chu's bill was the better of the two.

And Ms. Pratt and Mr. Leishman, if I could—saw your heads nodding in a firm agreement. Would you state if I was correct in saying that you agree that the Chu bill would be preferable? Please don't nod.

Ms. PRATT. So I—this is Ms. Pratt, and I do agree that the—Representative Chu's bill heads in the right direction. And I would add to that my comment that I think a group representing a variety of different perspectives, including the perspectives represented here at this table would be useful to inform a process.

Mr. COHEN. Thank you. Mr. Leishman.

Mr. LEISHMAN. I agree. Congresswoman Chu's bill is great. Congressman Rohrabacher's bill goes several steps too far, in my opinion. It is similar to, but not as good as, Congressman Issa's bill— I believe it was 472—and I highly endorse that bill.

Mr. COHEN. Thank you. And I am not going to put Mr. Peterson on the spot, because Dana is my friend, and I suspect Dana is your friend.

Mr. PETERSON. Yes, sir.

Mr. COHEN. Good, thank you.

I want to introduce on the record Mr. Nadler's statement, and a statement—a letter from the Consortium for Citizens with Disabilities. And I would like to——

Mr. KING. Without objection, so ordered. [The information follows:]

Mr. COHEN. And I would like to read my opening statement, and I am going to try to do that within the 3 minutes and 28 seconds. Today's hearing focused on Sober Living Homes, which are group homes for persons who are recovering from alcohol or substance addiction. In particular, it focused on whether the Fair Housing Act and Americans With Disabilities Act, and potentially other federal civil rights statutes need to be amended to allow state and localities to regulate sober homes.

I take no position on the question of whether sober homes are the best means of integrating those recovering from addiction in society, nor do I have a view as to what might constitute best practices regarding the operation of sober homes. Those questions are beyond the jurisdiction and expertise of this subcommittee.

As the subcommittee with jurisdiction over our Nation's civil rights laws, however, we must be very wary of attempts to create exemptions to such laws or otherwise weaken their enforcement mechanisms.

Both the Fair Housing Act and the ADA prohibit discrimination against persons with disabilities with respect to housing and persons recovering from alcohol or substance addiction are considered to be disabled, and therefore, entitled to protections under those statutes. Congress passed these laws in order to counteract the effects of generations of stigma, negative stereotypes, social societal prejudice to keep persons with disabilities segregated and isolated from mainstream society.

As a person with a disability, I am sensitive to any attempt to weaken these protections for these laws. I share the goal of ensuring that persons with disabilities are able to integrate and participate fully in the important aspect of American life: namely, the chance to live in a residential area among members of the broader society.

Some municipalities claim they are too afraid to regulate Sober Living Homes because they fear being sued for violating the Fair Housing Act or the ADA. And indeed, cities have been sued successfully for violating those laws using zoning or land use regulations to restrict Sober Living Homes. Therefore, they seek an exemption to these statutes with respect to the regulation of Sober Living Homes.

The fact is, however, that Sober Living Homes can be regulated without creating carve-outs to the civil rights laws. Indeed, group homes that serve persons with other types of disabilities are already regulated by states and localities without any need for a special exemption from the Fair Housing Act or the ADA. There is no reason Sober Living Homes cannot similarly be regulated within the existing confines of those statutes.

Towards the end of the Obama Administration the Department of Justice and Department of Housing and Urban Development issued updated guidance answering specific questions commonly asked by states and localities about how to apply zoning and land use laws in ways that do not violate the Fair Housing Act. This guidance, in turn, updated previous long-standing guidance issued in the 1999—governing group homes and the Fair Housing Act.

Moreover, the Fair Housing Act itself allows considerable flexibility for cities to address some of the very real abuses that sometimes occur with respect to the operation of for-profit Sober Living Homes. For instance, it would not violate the statute to deny housing to someone who would constitute a direct threat to the health or safety of others, or would result in substantial property damage. Also, it does not permit discrimination complaints by those who currently use a controlled substance.

I recognize there are legitimate concerns with the conduct of some Sober Living Home operators. Those who engage in fraud and abuse of residents can and should be punished, and reasonable regulation can and should be adopted.

And I didn't know about the Florida Triangle, but that is shocking, that people do that.

Doing so, however, does not require exemptions to civil rights law. The prior legislative proposals to do so dating back to the 1990s have all died in committee, and rightly so.

I appreciate the witnesses for coming here, I apologize for being late. I am a big fan of Judy's, and I am a big fan of Dana's. So I appreciate them being here, and may God save the United States of America.

Mr. COHEN. I yield back the balance of my time.

Mr. KING. The chair thanks the gentleman, the ranking member from Tennessee.

And now I will recognize the gentleman from Florida, Mr. Deutch.

Mr. DEUTCH. Thank you, Mr. Chairman, and thanks to all of our witnesses for being here today.

Mr. Chairman, we have, as Mr. Aronberg pointed out, a lot of experience with sober homes in Florida. And to that end I ask unanimous consent to enter three letters that convey that experience from the City of Delray Beach, Florida; the City of Coconut Creek, Florida; and the Florida Association of Recovery Residences. I ask that they be entered into the record this morning.

Mr. KING. Without objection, so ordered. [The information follows:]

Mr. DEUTCH. Thank you, Mr. Chairman. In Florida, an average day means that 15 people die from an overdose. It is tragic, it is unacceptable, and we have got to do everything we can to stop it. We have to help Americans find sobriety and maintain recovery. We have to try to save lives.

Addiction is not about weak families, it is about a disease. And I would just point out that, because it is a disease, it is in our best interests to ensure that we do everything we can to help people get care, which is why the idea of repealing the Affordable Care Act and costing 2.8 million people with substance use disorders their access to health care, and 220,000 with opioid disorders losing their access would be an enormous step backward.

There is a battle and a war on overdose, and we have to end the stigma of addiction. Ending the federal housing protections won't win that battle. It is not theoretical. People with mental illness and substance abuse disorder suffer discrimination every day.

A 2017 study by the Department of Housing and Urban Development found that people with mental illnesses face serious barriers in their search for a home. Improper requests to disclose personal and disability-related information steering toward specific housing, based on the individual's disabilities [sic].

The Fair Housing Act was not, however, intended to protect businesses who take advantage of people struggling with substance use disorders to line their own pockets. So we can stop bad actors who encourage relapse and overdose and protect our communities, while maintaining discrimination protections at the same time. We can do both. Ms. Pratt talked about that, Mr. Aronberg talked about that.

Mr. Aronberg, I am proud to have you here today to share your work with the committee. And I would note that you appeared before the Energy and Commerce Committee of this House last December. Your testimony and the testimony of Assistant State Attorney Al Johnson was instrumental in the creation of legislation that supported information—legislation that was included in the final opioids legislation that this House will vote on in about an hour. That bill will make it illegal to pay kickbacks for getting people in the door at sober homes and clinics. So you have already helped advance federal efforts to stop these abuses, and we are grateful for that.

What I would like to know—you started touching on this—you talked about reissuing—the joint statement, you talked about reasonable standards and model criteria. Tell us how that can be helpful. Tell us how what we are doing today, together with those efforts, can help to stop the schemes that you described and showed on the slides.

Mr. ARONBERG. Thank you, Congressman Deutch, and thank you for your nice words. I really appreciate it.

As you can see from this panel, we come from different communities and different backgrounds. You could say different perspectives on this. But we seem to agree that you can work within the existing laws by clarifying them to really help fix a lot of these problems. And we may differ as to degree, but there—I think there is a consensus on that. And one way to do it is through the joint clarification.

There was a joint statement issued by HUD and DOJ in December of 2016 that, in talking to local governments in Florida, wasn't very clarifying. It wasn't very helpful. And I can tell you from our law enforcement perspective, it has not been very helpful.

And I think that you may not even have to rewrite it, you can just add a 17th question. There were 16 questions and answers, and the 17th—and I have provided a sample in my written remarks, which allow local governments to implement licensing and reasonable regulations that are narrowly tailored to meet the actual needs of the occupants in recovery. And I think that would be consistent with the ADA and the FHA.

And you asked about what other communities are doing. In Delray Beach, which is in your district, or used to be in your district, actually, before the reapportionment, in order—they have a new ordinance there that, in order to obtain a reasonable accommodation, which is for more than three unrelated adults in Delray Beach, that the house, the sober home, needs to be certified or otherwise demonstrate adherence to recognize national standards. And there is two ways to do that: through NARR, National Association of Recovery Residences and its affiliate, FARR, which have nationally recognized standards; or through an Oxford House model. And so this is the way that Delray Beach is doing it.

Now, one reason why I am here, and I think others are here, is because local governments such as Huntington Beach are afraid to do what Delray Beach did because they could get sued. Delray Beach is doing it. They haven't been sued yet. But that is why the Federal Government needs to give more clarification to local governments, to let them know.

Can they do what Delray Beach did? Can they act in this way? I think they can, but right now local governments are going out there on their own, and we need to give them a little more protection and clarification.

Mr. DEUTCH. Mr. Chairman, this is a really important topic, and I appreciate your holding this hearing. And it means a great deal that the witnesses made time to be here, as——

Mr. KING. The gentleman is granted unanimous consent for an additional minute.

Mr. DEUTCH. No, I am through, Mr. Chairman. Thank you. It was just to express my thanks to you for holding this hearing.

Mr. KING. Okay, I appreciate that. And I want to express my gratitude to all the witnesses here this morning. And this concludes today's hearing.

And without objection, all members will have five legislative days to submit additional written questions for the witnesses or additional materials for the record.

I thank each of you, and this hearing is now adjourned. [Whereupon, at 10:07 a.m., the Subcommittee was adjourned.]

INDEX

B

C

L

M

N

O

P

Q

R

S

T

U

V

W

Y